DISCARD

MedMaps for
Pathophysiology

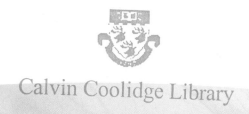

MedMaps for
Pathophysiology

Yasmeen Agosti

Drexel University College of Medicine, Class of 2008
Philadelphia, Pennsylvania

Pamela Duke, MD

Assistant Professor of Medicine
Division of General Internal Medicine
Course Director Pathophysiology and Clinical Skills, Program for Integrated Learning
Drexel University College of Medicine
Philadelphia, Pennsylvania

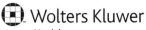 Wolters Kluwer | Lippincott Williams & Wilkins
Health
Philadelphia • Baltimore • New York • London
Buenos Aires • Hong Kong • Sydney • Tokyo

Acquisitions Editor: Nancy Duffy
Developmental Editor: Kathleen H. Scogna
Marketing Manager: Emilie Moyer
Sales Representative: John Friscia
Production Editor: Gina Aiello
Art Director: Doug Smock
Compositor: International Typesetting and Composition
Printer: Data Reproduction Corp.

Library of Congress Cataloging-in-Publication Data

Agosti, Yasmeen.
    MedMaps for pathophysiology / Yasmeen Agosti, Pamela Duke.
        p. ; cm.
    Includes bibliographical references and index.
    ISBN-13: 978-0-7817-7755-1
    ISBN-10: 0-7817-7755-0
1. Pathology.   I. Duke, Pamela.   II. Title.
    [DNLM: 1. Pathology.   QZ 4 A275m 2008]
    RB111.M4387 2008
    616.07—dc22

                            2007008897

In memory of a dear friend and colleague Steven Charles Boyle, DUCOM class of 2007, who would have made an excellent emergency medicine physician.

Pathophysiology can be a challenging subject to master because of its interdisciplinary nature. The course is traditionally taught in the second year of medical school and should be seen as a bridge from the basic sciences in the first two years to clinical practice during the clerkships and beyond. Each year as students are required to learn more and more material, the goal of developing clinical reasoning skills becomes overshadowed by the volume of detail. Consequently, many textbooks used by medical students often feel overloaded with basic science or, alternatively, too advanced in terms of diagnosis and management. *MedMaps for Pathophysiology* aims to strike a balance between basic concepts, disease processes, and the clinical approach.

The purpose of this book is to introduce the concept map as an alternative format for understanding pathophysiology. *MedMaps* allows for both understanding disease mechanisms and remembering them in a visually meaningful way. Each map takes its own individual shape, and it is our hope that this will help the visual learner to master disease processes. By design, the maps allow the student to add details from lectures or readings so that they can begin to own the ideas rather than just memorizing them. Ultimately, the maps become a customized reference as personal notes and clinical experiences reinforce the understanding of the disease process. This is a book that can accompany students throughout their years in medical school as they transition from learning to practicing medicine.

The disease topics in this book are organized by organ system. As this approach is used in many larger medical textbooks, *MedMaps* will be easy to use alongside a larger resource. Within each organ system are disease topics, which are most likely to be encountered in the classroom, on board exams, and in the clinical setting. The disease process begins at the top of the page with etiologies or triggering mechanisms and then makes its way down the page to clinical presentation. Along the way, we have carefully chosen the most relevant details as appropriate for the level of second-year medical students. The flow of the arrows is meant to guide the reader through interconnecting details which may not be as obvious in the form of traditional paragraph text. Shared endpoints such as "heart failure" or "anemia" are referenced to maps on other pages so that the reader is able to see larger connections amidst the finer detail. A blank page to the left of each map is provided for additional note taking as the student's knowledge base evolves. Several "general" maps such as "coagulation cascade" and "cell-mediated immunity" have also been provided to supplement many disease states, which share a common physiological mechanism. An index in the back references key words found within the maps, as well as the actual names of diseases, to facilitate the use of this book.

We hope that you enjoy using *MedMaps for Pathophysiology* and we welcome your input for future editions.

MedMaps KEY	
hatch mark	denotes point in disease process where abnormality or dysfunction occurs (for example Hypocalcemia map)
dotted line	designates portion of map that describes pathophysiology in relation to a normal process (for example Cushing's map)
boxed items	used to call attention to a detail in the disease process
bolded text	used to call attention to a key detail in the disease process
"see map"	refers to another map with which pathophysiology overlaps or connects
⇩ ⇧	denotes "decrease" and "increase"

ACKNOWLEDGMENTS

My biggest and most important thank you goes to my husband Alex and my son Paolo for being the total joy of my life. I would also like to thank my parents for providing me with a rich education both inside and outside the classroom. Finally, I would like to thank my coauthor Pam Duke, who not only made this book project a truly enjoyable collaboration but has also shown me how to be both a physician and a human being at the same time.

-Yaz M. Agosti

I would not have been able to do this if not for the support and constant inspiration of my husband Laurent. Many thanks go to my three patients and wonderful children Alexandre, Mireille, and Natasha. I would like to thank my coauthor Yaz Agosti for her initiative and creativity throughout this project. My inspiration for going into medicine is from my father, Martin Duke, who initially took me into the hospital and whose own intellectual curiosity instilled in me a desire to pursue academic medicine. And the initial strength to persevere is from my mother, Juliane Duke, whose spirit is in everything I do.

-Pamela Duke

We both would like to thank the following individuals for their support: Marcello Malakooti for his many insights and encouragements, Dr. James England, Dr. Burton Landau, Dr. Cheryl Hanau, Dr. Samuel Parrish, Dr. Kristen Larson, the Program for Integrated Learning spearheaded by Dr. Charles Puglia, Dr. Sue Zern, Dr. Thad Wilson, Donna Boyle, Qing Li, Randi Leigh, Danielle Press, Irene Mason, and the Drexel library staff at the Queen Lane campus. We would also like to thank several people at LWW without whom this book would not have been possible – Betty Sun, Kathleen Scogna, Nancy Duffy, Nicole Williams, and John Frisca.

CONTENTS

General Maps

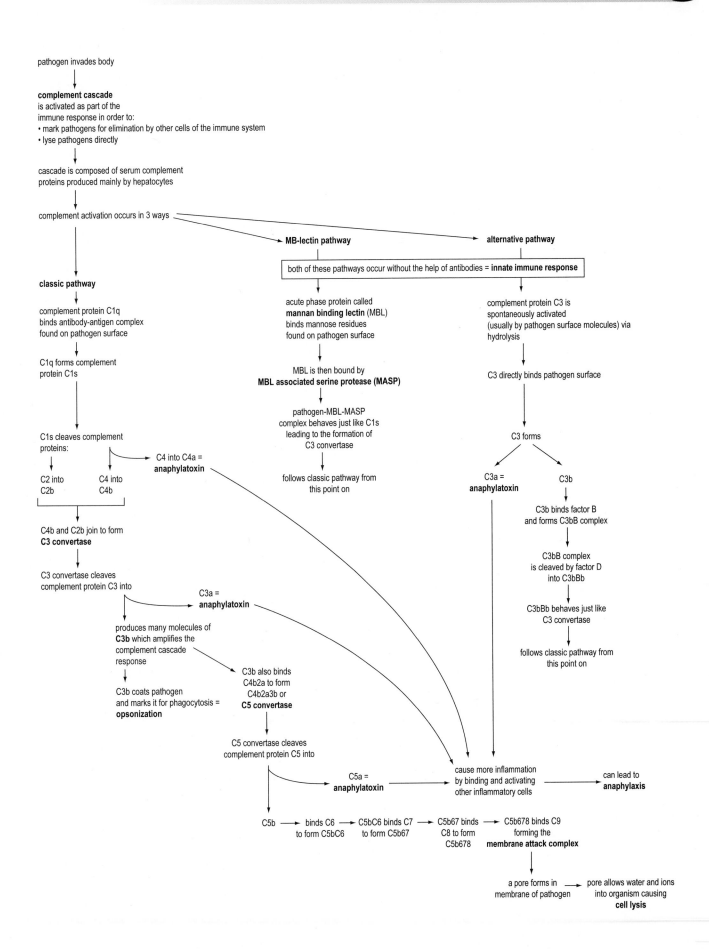

pathogen invades body

complement cascade
is activated as part of the
immune response in order to:
• mark pathogens for elimination by other cells of the immune system
• lyse pathogens directly

cascade is composed of serum complement
proteins produced mainly by hepatocytes

complement activation occurs in 3 ways

MB-lectin pathway

alternative pathway

both of these pathways occur without the help of antibodies = **innate immune response**

classic pathway

complement protein C1q
binds antibody-antigen complex
found on pathogen surface

C1q forms complement
protein C1s

C1s cleaves complement
proteins:

C2 into
C2b

C4 into
C4b

C4 into C4a =
anaphylatoxin

C4b and C2b join to form
C3 convertase

C3 convertase cleaves
complement protein C3 into

C3a =
anaphylatoxin

produces many molecules of
C3b which amplifies the
complement cascade
response

C3b coats pathogen
and marks it for phagocytosis =
opsonization

C3b also binds
C4b2a to form
C4b2a3b or
C5 convertase

C5 convertase cleaves
complement protein C5 into

C5a =
anaphylatoxin

acute phase protein called
mannan binding lectin (MBL)
binds mannose residues
found on pathogen surface

MBL is then bound by
MBL associated serine protease (MASP)

pathogen-MBL-MASP
complex behaves just like C1s
leading to the formation of
C3 convertase

follows classic pathway from
this point on

complement protein C3 is
spontaneously activated
(usually by pathogen surface molecules) via
hydrolysis

C3 directly binds pathogen surface

C3 forms

C3a =
anaphylatoxin

C3b

C3b binds factor B
and forms C3bB complex

C3bB complex
is cleaved by factor D
into C3bBb

C3bBb behaves just like
C3 convertase

follows classic pathway from
this point on

cause more inflammation
by binding and activating
other inflammatory cells

can lead to
anaphylaxis

C5b ⟶ binds C6
to form C5bC6 ⟶ C5bC6 binds C7
to form C5b67 ⟶ C5b67 binds
C8 to form
C5b678 ⟶ C5b678 binds C9
forming the
membrane attack complex

a pore forms in
membrane of pathogen ⟶ pore allows water and ions
into organism causing
cell lysis

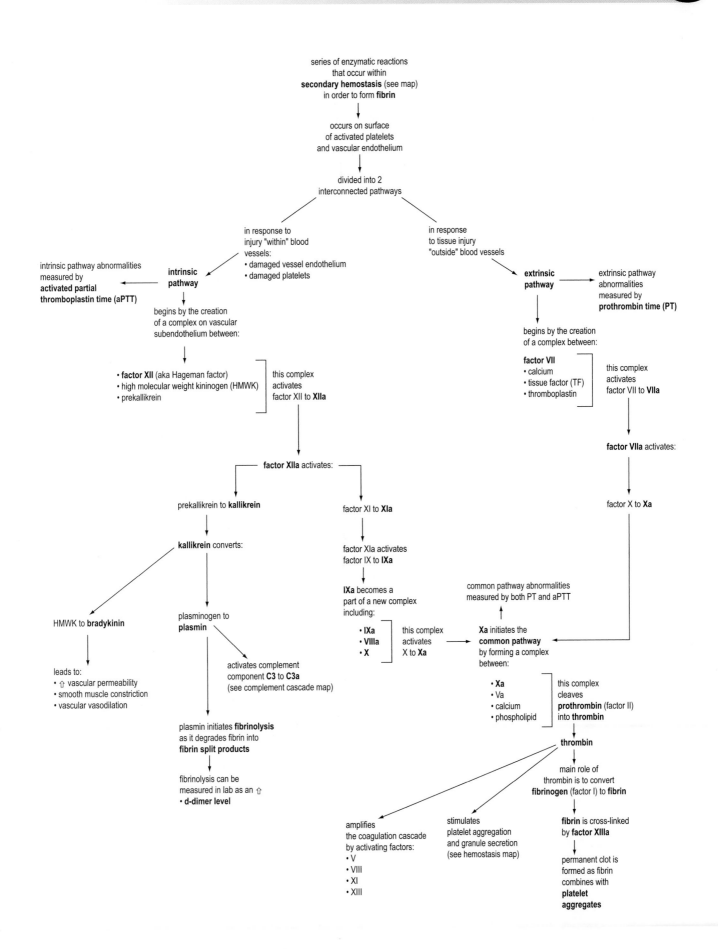

series of enzymatic reactions
that occur within
secondary hemostasis (see map)
in order to form **fibrin**

occurs on surface
of activated platelets
and vascular endothelium

divided into 2
interconnected pathways

in response to
injury "within" blood
vessels:
• damaged vessel endothelium
• damaged platelets

in response
to tissue injury
"outside" blood vessels

intrinsic pathway abnormalities
measured by
**activated partial
thromboplastin time (aPTT)**

**intrinsic
pathway**

begins by the creation
of a complex on vascular
subendothelium between:

• **factor XII** (aka Hageman factor)
• high molecular weight kininogen (HMWK)
• prekallikrein

this complex
activates
factor XII to **XIIa**

factor XIIa activates:

prekallikrein to **kallikrein**

factor XI to **XIa**

factor XIa activates
factor IX to **IXa**

kallikrein converts:

IXa becomes a
part of a new complex
including:

common pathway abnormalities
measured by both PT and aPTT

HMWK to **bradykinin**

plasminogen to
plasmin

• **IXa**
• **VIIIa**
• **X**

this complex
activates
X to **Xa**

Xa initiates the
common pathway
by forming a complex
between:

leads to:
• ⇧ vascular permeability
• smooth muscle constriction
• vascular vasodilation

activates complement
component **C3** to **C3a**
(see complement cascade map)

• **Xa**
• Va
• calcium
• phospholipid

this complex
cleaves
prothrombin (factor II)
into **thrombin**

plasmin initiates **fibrinolysis**
as it degrades fibrin into
fibrin split products

thrombin

fibrinolysis can be
measured in lab as an ⇧
• **d-dimer level**

main role of
thrombin is to convert
fibrinogen (factor I) to **fibrin**

amplifies
the coagulation cascade
by activating factors:
• V
• VIII
• XI
• XIII

stimulates
platelet aggregation
and granule secretion
(see hemostasis map)

fibrin is cross-linked
by **factor XIIIa**

permanent clot is
formed as fibrin
combines with
**platelet
aggregates**

**extrinsic
pathway**

extrinsic pathway
abnormalities
measured by
prothrombin time (PT)

begins by the creation
of a complex between:

factor VII
• calcium
• tissue factor (TF)
• thromboplastin

this complex
activates
factor VII to **VIIa**

factor VIIa activates:

factor X to **Xa**

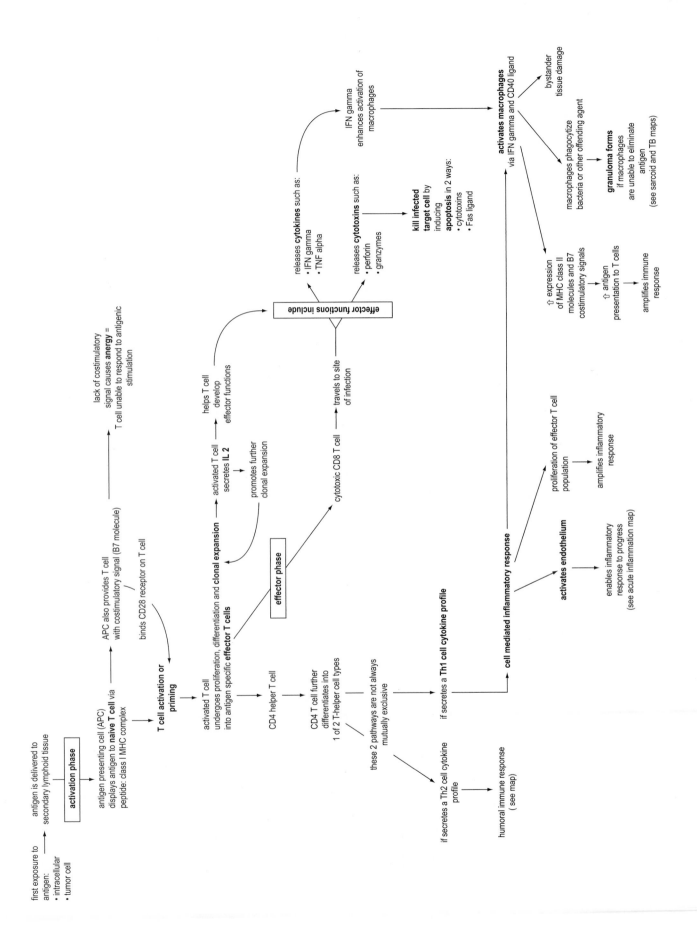

first exposure to antigen:
• intracellular
• tumor cell

antigen is delivered to secondary lymphoid tissue

activation phase

antigen presenting cell (APC) displays antigen to **naive T cell** via peptide: class I MHC complex

APC also provides T cell with costimulatory signal (B7 molecule)

binds CD28 receptor on T cell

lack of costimulatory signal causes **anergy** = T cell unable to respond to antigenic stimulation

T cell activation or priming

activated T cell undergoes proliferation, differentiation and **clonal expansion** into antigen specific **effector T cells**

CD4 helper T cell

CD4 T cell further differentiates into 1 of 2 T-helper cell types

these 2 pathways are not always mutually exclusive

if secretes a Th2 cell cytokine profile

humoral immune response (see map)

if secretes a **Th1 cell cytokine profile**

cell mediated inflammatory response

activated T cell secretes **IL 2**

promotes further clonal expansion

helps T cell develop effector functions

effector phase

cytotoxic CD8 T cell ⟶ travels to site of infection

effector functions include

releases **cytokines** such as:
• IFN gamma
• TNF alpha

IFN gamma enhances activation of macrophages

releases **cytotoxins** such as:
• perforin
• granzymes

kill infected target cell by inducing **apoptosis** in 2 ways:
• cytotoxins
• Fas ligand

activates macrophages
via IFN gamma and CD40 ligand

bystander tissue damage

macrophages phagocytize bacteria or other offending agent

granuloma forms
if macrophages are unable to eliminate antigen
(see sarcoid and TB maps)

⇧ expression of MHC class II molecules and B7 costimulatory signals

⇧ antigen presentation to T cells

amplifies immune response

activates endothelium

proliferation of effector T cell population

amplifies inflammatory response

enables inflammatory response to progress (see acute inflammation map)

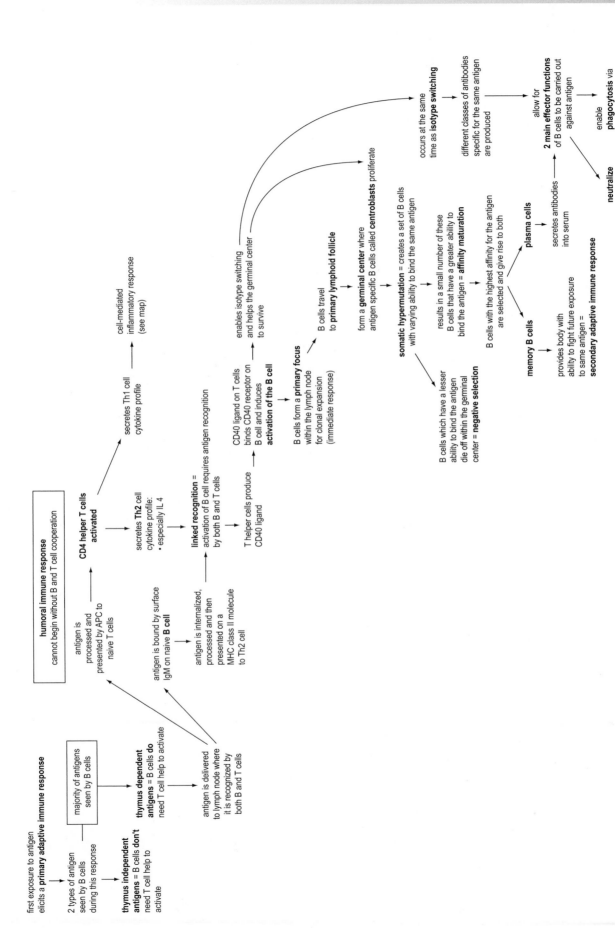

first exposure to antigen
elicits a **primary adaptive immune response**

2 types of antigen
seen by B cells
during this response

**thymus independent
antigens** = B cells **don't**
need T cell help to
activate

majority of antigens
seen by B cells

**thymus dependent
antigens** = B cells **do**
need T cell help to activate

antigen is delivered
to lymph node where
it is recognized by
both B and T cells

humoral immune response
cannot begin without B and T cell cooperation

antigen is
processed and
presented by APC to
naive T cells

antigen is bound by surface
IgM on naive **B cell**

antigen is internalized,
processed and then
presented on a
MHC class II molecule
to Th2 cell

**CD4 helper T cells
activated**

secretes Th1 cell
cytokine profile

cell-mediated
inflammatory response
(see map)

secretes **Th2** cell
cytokine profile:
• especially IL 4

linked recognition =
activation of B cell requires antigen recognition
by both B and T cells

T helper cells produce
CD40 ligand

CD40 ligand on T cells
binds CD40 receptor on
B cell and induces
activation of the B cell

B cells form a **primary focus**
within the lymph node
for clonal expansion
(immediate response)

enables isotype switching
and helps the germinal center
to survive

B cells travel
to **primary lymphoid follicle**

form a **germinal center** where
antigen specific B cells called **centroblasts** proliferate

somatic hypermutation = creates a set of B cells
with varying ability to bind the same antigen

B cells which have a lesser
ability to bind the antigen
die off within the germinal
center = **negative selection**

results in a small number of these
B cells that have a greater ability to
bind the antigen = **affinity maturation**

B cells with the highest affinity for the antigen
are selected and give rise to both

plasma cells

memory B cells

occurs at the same
time as **isotype switching**

different classes of antibodies
specific for the same antigen
are produced

secretes antibodies
into serum

provides body with
ability to fight future exposure
to same antigen =
secondary adaptive immune response

allow for
2 main effector functions
of B cells to be carried out
against antigen

**neutralize
pathogens** =
binding and preventing
pathogens from
entering cells

enable
phagocytosis via
2 ways:
• opsonization
• complement
  activation (see map)

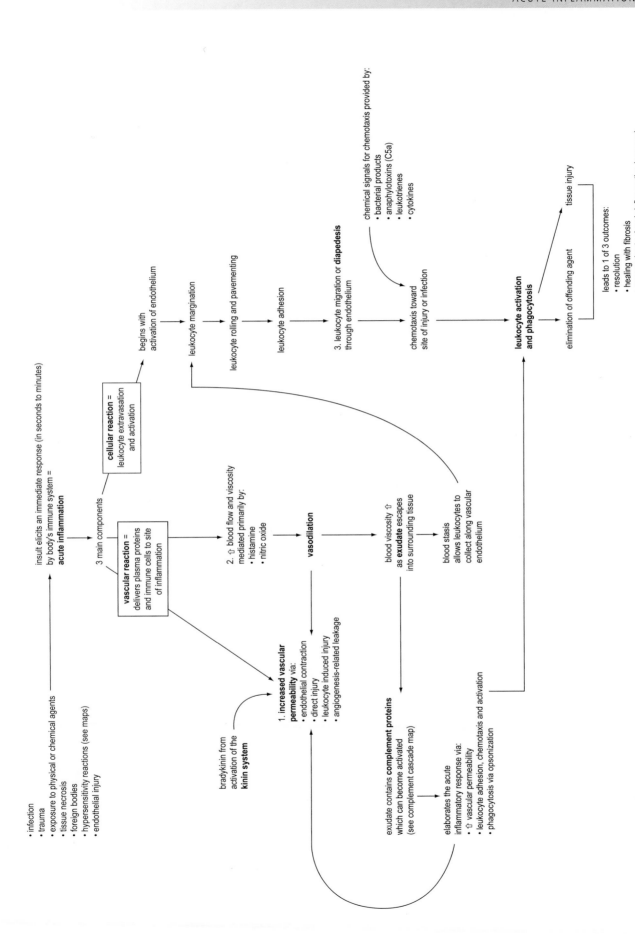

- infection
- trauma
- exposure to physical or chemical agents
- tissue necrosis
- foreign bodies
- hypersensitivity reactions (see maps)
- endothelial injury

insult elicits an immediate response (in seconds to minutes) by body's immune system = **acute inflammation**

3 main components

cellular reaction = leukocyte extravasation and activation

vascular reaction = delivers plasma proteins and immune cells to site of inflammation

begins with activation of endothelium

leukocyte margination

leukocyte rolling and pavementing

leukocyte adhesion

3. leukocyte migration or **diapedesis** through endothelium

chemical signals for chemotaxis provided by:
- bacterial products
- anaphylotoxins (C5a)
- leukotrienes
- cytokines

chemotaxis toward site of injury or infection

leukocyte activation and phagocytosis

elimination of offending agent

tissue injury

leads to 1 of 3 outcomes:
- resolution
- healing with fibrosis
- progression to chronic inflammation (see map)

2. ⇧ blood flow and viscosity mediated primarily by:
- histamine
- nitric oxide

vasodilation

blood viscosity ⇧ as **exudate** escapes into surrounding tissue

blood stasis allows leukocytes to collect along vascular endothelium

1. **increased vascular permeability** via:
- endothelial contraction
- direct injury
- leukocyte induced injury
- angiogenesis-related leakage

bradykinin from activation of the **kinin system**

exudate contains **complement proteins** which can become activated (see complement cascade map)

elaborates the acute inflammatory response via:
- ⇧ vascular permeability
- leukocyte adhesion, chemotaxis and activation
- phagocytosis via opsonization

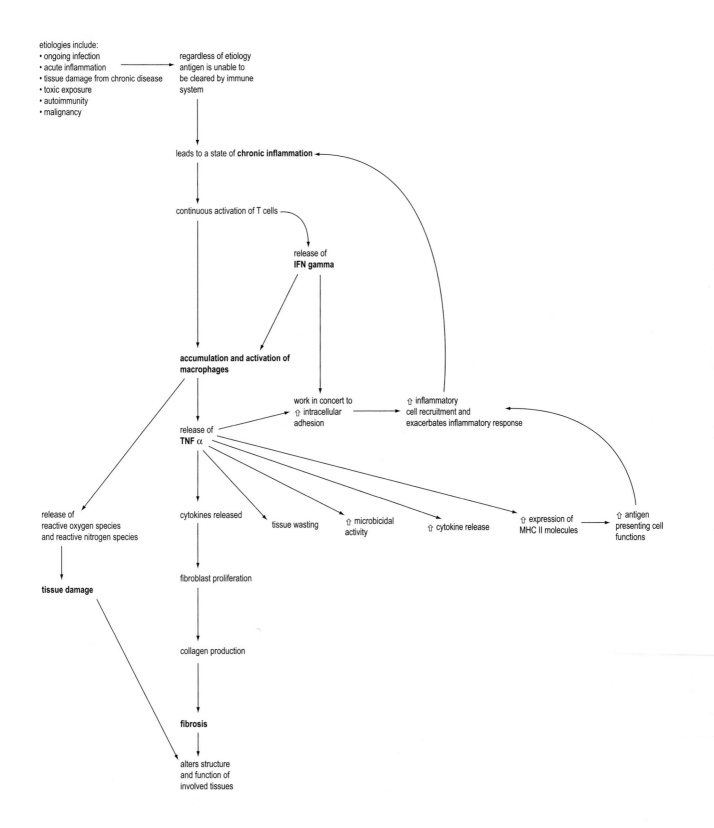

etiologies include:
- ongoing infection
- acute inflammation
- tissue damage from chronic disease
- toxic exposure
- autoimmunity
- malignancy

regardless of etiology antigen is unable to be cleared by immune system

leads to a state of **chronic inflammation**

continuous activation of T cells

release of **IFN gamma**

accumulation and activation of macrophages

work in concert to ⇧ intracellular adhesion

⇧ inflammatory cell recruitment and exacerbates inflammatory response

release of **TNF α**

release of reactive oxygen species and reactive nitrogen species

cytokines released

tissue wasting

⇧ microbicidal activity

⇧ cytokine release

⇧ expression of MHC II molecules

⇧ antigen presenting cell functions

tissue damage

fibroblast proliferation

collagen production

fibrosis

alters structure and function of involved tissues

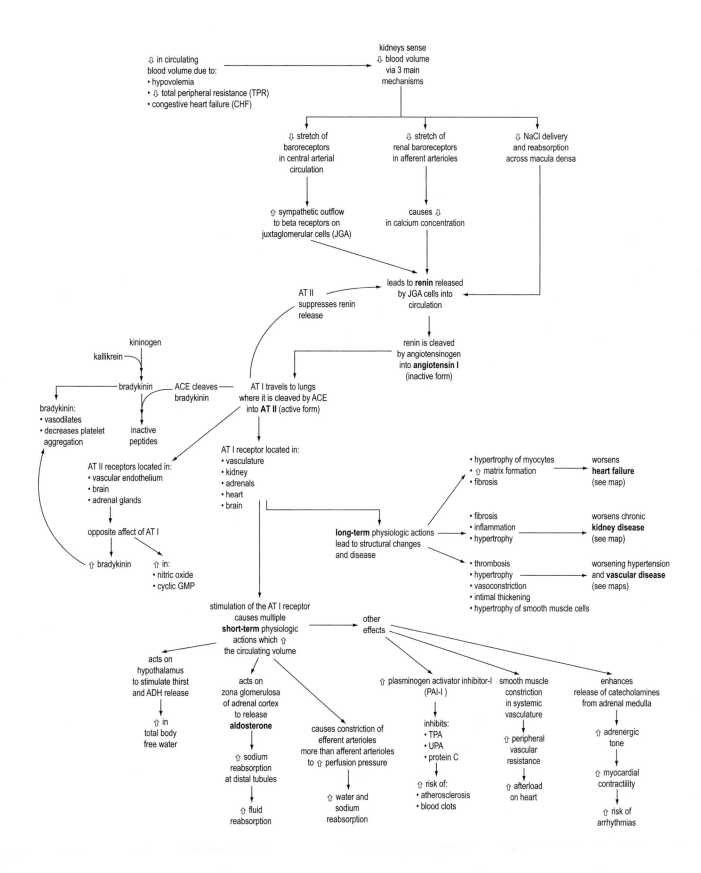

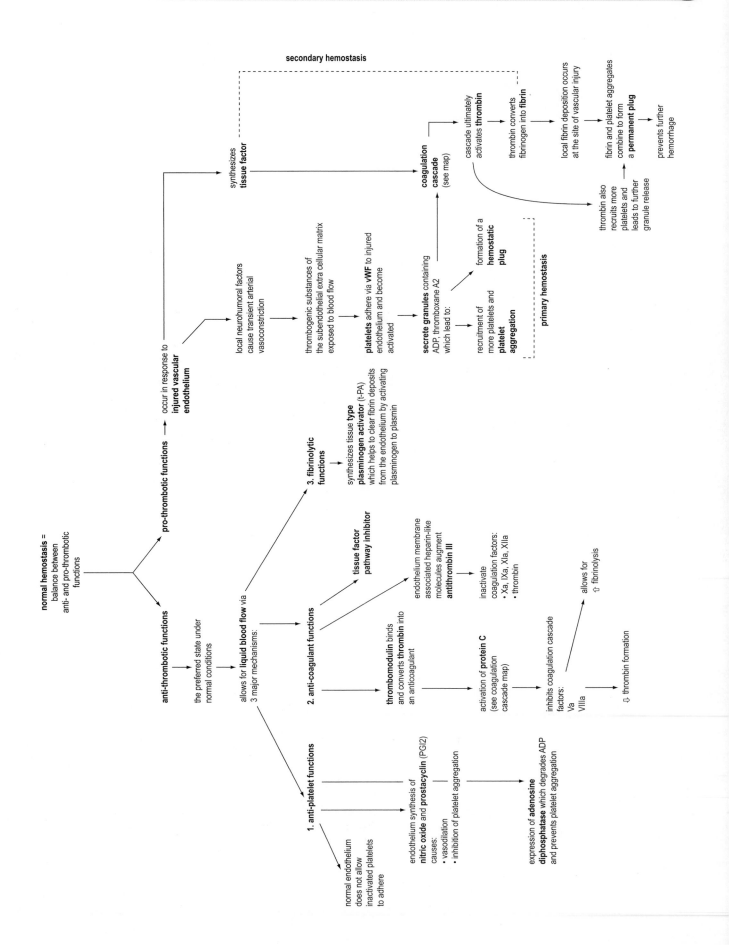

secondary hemostasis

synthesizes **tissue factor**

occur in response to **injured vascular endothelium**

local neurohumoral factors cause transient arterial vasoconstriction

thrombogenic substances of the subendothelial extra cellular matrix exposed to blood flow

platelets adhere via **vWF** to injured endothelium and become activated

secrete granules containing ADP, thromboxane A2 which lead to:

formation of a **hemostatic plug**

recruitment of more platelets and **platelet aggregation**

primary hemostasis

coagulation cascade (see map)

cascade ultimately activates **thrombin**

thrombin converts fibrinogen into **fibrin**

local fibrin deposition occurs at the site of vascular injury

fibrin and platelet aggregates combine to form a **permanent plug**

prevents further hemorrhage

thrombin also recruits more platelets and leads to further granule release

pro-thrombotic functions

normal hemostasis = balance between anti- and pro-thrombotic functions

anti-thrombotic functions

the preferred state under normal conditions

allows for **liquid blood flow** via 3 major mechanisms:

3. fibrinolytic functions

synthesizes tissue **type plasminogen activator** (t-PA) which helps to clear fibrin deposits from the endothelium by activating plasminogen to plasmin

2. anti-coagulant functions

tissue factor pathway inhibitor

endothelium membrane associated heparin-like molecules augment **antithrombin III**

inactivate coagulation factors:
• Xa, IXa, XIa, XIIa
• thrombin

thrombomodulin binds and converts **thrombin** into an anticoagulant

activation of **protein C** (see coagulation cascade map)

inhibits coagulation cascade factors:
Va
VIIIa

allows for ⇑ fibrinolysis

⇓ thrombin formation

1. anti-platelet functions

normal endothelium does not allow inactivated platelets to adhere

endothelium synthesis of **nitric oxide** and **prostacyclin** (PGI2) causes:
• vasodilation
• inhibition of platelet aggregation

expression of **adenosine diphosphatase** which degrades ADP and prevents platelet aggregation

Cardiovascular Disorders

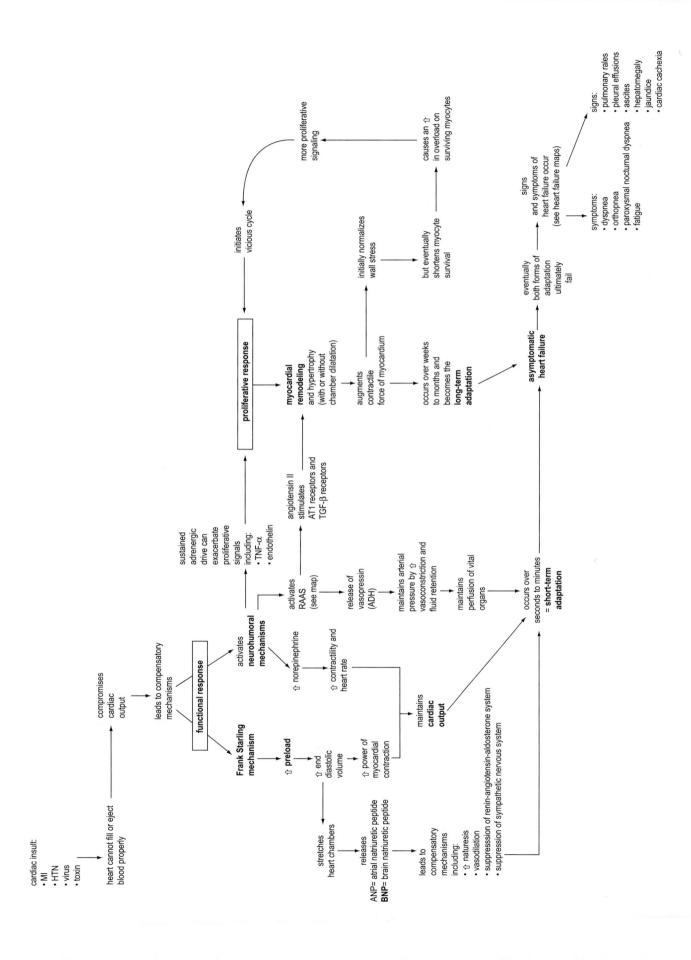

cardiac insult:
• MI
• HTN
• virus
• toxin

heart cannot fill or eject blood properly → compromises cardiac output → leads to compensatory mechanisms

functional response

activates **neurohumoral mechanisms**

Frank Starling mechanism

⇧ **preload** → ⇧ end diastolic volume → ⇧ power of myocardial contraction → maintains **cardiac output**

⇧ norepinephrine → ⇧ contractility and heart rate

stretches heart chambers → releases

ANP= atrial natriuretic peptide
BNP= brain natriuretic peptide

leads to compensatory mechanisms including:
• ⇧ natriuresis
• vasodilation
• suppresssion of renin-angiotensin-aldosterone system
• suppression of sympathetic nervous system

activates RAAS (see map) → release of vasopressin (ADH) → maintains arterial pressure by ⇧ vasoconstriction and fluid retention → maintains perfusion of vital organs → occurs over seconds to minutes = **short-term adaptation**

sustained adrenergic drive can exacerbate proliferative signals including:
• TNF-α
• endothelin

angiotensin II stimulates AT1 receptors and TGF-β receptors

proliferative response

initiates vicious cycle

more proliferative signaling

myocardial remodeling and hypertrophy (with or without chamber dilatation)

initially normalizes wall stress

augments contractile force of myocardium

but eventually shortens myocyte survival

causes an ⇧ in overload on surviving myocytes

occurs over weeks to months and becomes the **long-term adaptation**

asymptomatic heart failure

eventually both forms of adaptation ultimately fail

signs and symptoms of heart failure occur (see heart failure maps)

symptoms:
• dyspnea
• orthopnea
• paroxysmal nocturnal dyspnea
• fatigue

signs:
• pulmonary rales
• pleural effusions
• ascites
• hepatomegaly
• jaundice
• cardiac cachexia

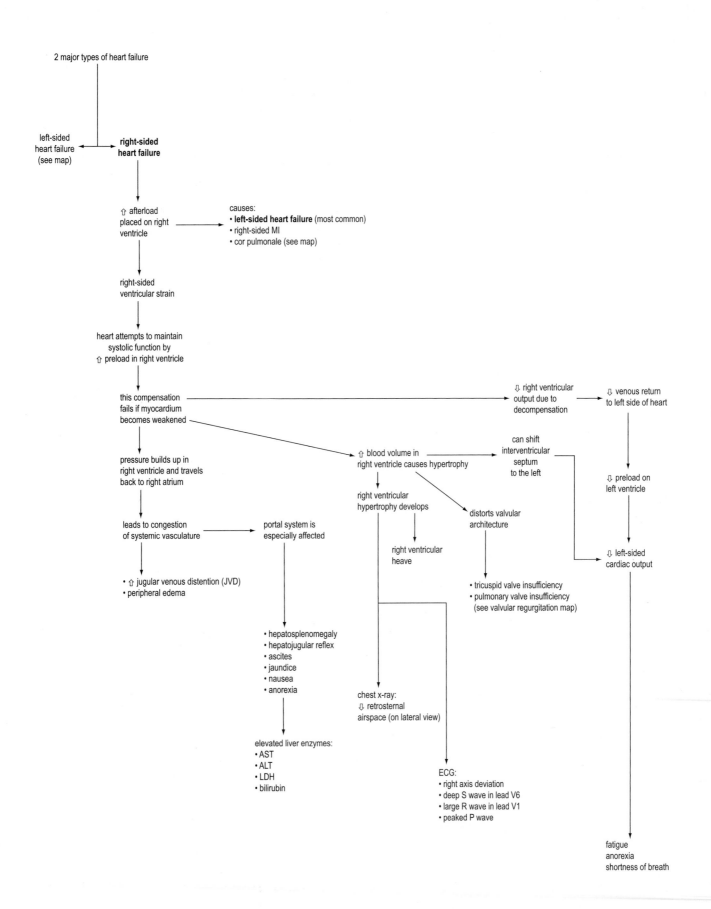

2 major types of heart failure

left-sided
heart failure
(see map)

**right-sided
heart failure**

⇧ afterload
placed on right
ventricle

causes:
• **left-sided heart failure** (most common)
• right-sided MI
• cor pulmonale (see map)

right-sided
ventricular strain

heart attempts to maintain
systolic function by
⇧ preload in right ventricle

this compensation
fails if myocardium
becomes weakened

⇩ right ventricular
output due to
decompensation

⇩ venous return
to left side of heart

pressure builds up in
right ventricle and travels
back to right atrium

⇧ blood volume in
right ventricle causes hypertrophy

can shift
interventricular
septum
to the left

⇩ preload on
left ventricle

right ventricular
hypertrophy develops

distorts valvular
architecture

leads to congestion
of systemic vasculature

portal system is
especially affected

right ventricular
heave

⇩ left-sided
cardiac output

• ⇧ jugular venous distention (JVD)
• peripheral edema

• tricuspid valve insufficiency
• pulmonary valve insufficiency
  (see valvular regurgitation map)

• hepatosplenomegaly
• hepatojugular reflex
• ascites
• jaundice
• nausea
• anorexia

chest x-ray:
⇩ retrosternal
airspace (on lateral view)

elevated liver enzymes:
• AST
• ALT
• LDH
• bilirubin

ECG:
• right axis deviation
• deep S wave in lead V6
• large R wave in lead V1
• peaked P wave

fatigue
anorexia
shortness of breath

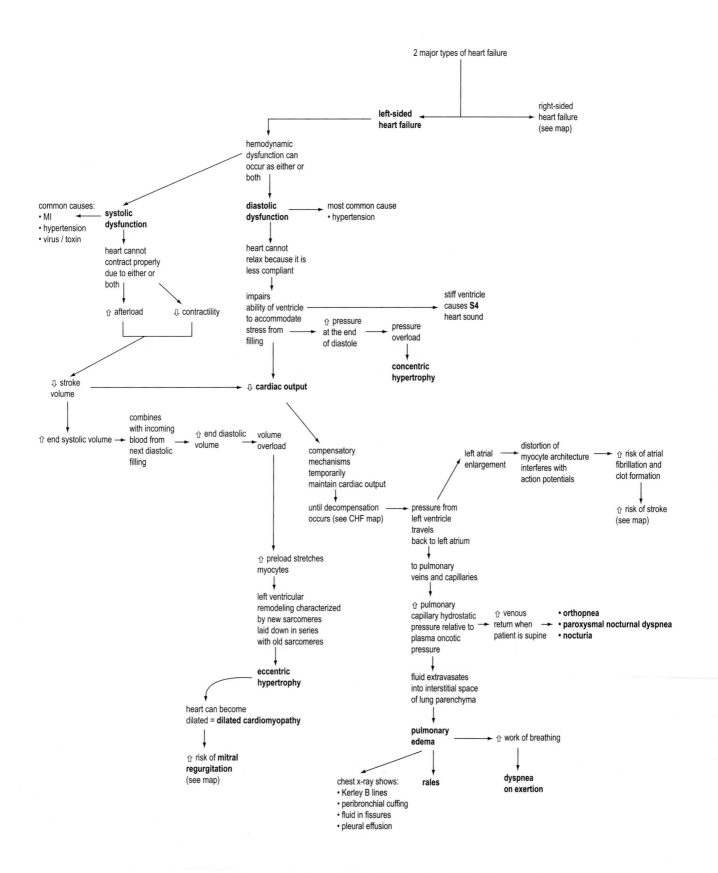

2 major types of heart failure

left-sided heart failure ← → right-sided heart failure (see map)

hemodynamic dysfunction can occur as either or both

common causes:
• MI
• hypertension
• virus / toxin

systolic dysfunction

diastolic dysfunction → most common cause • hypertension

heart cannot contract properly due to either or both

heart cannot relax because it is less compliant

⇧ afterload   ⇩ contractility

impairs ability of ventricle to accommodate stress from filling

stiff ventricle causes **S4** heart sound

⇧ pressure at the end of diastole → pressure overload

concentric hypertrophy

⇩ stroke volume

⇩ **cardiac output**

⇧ end systolic volume → combines with incoming blood from next diastolic filling → ⇧ end diastolic volume → volume overload

compensatory mechanisms temporarily maintain cardiac output

left atrial enlargement → distortion of myocyte architecture interferes with action potentials → ⇧ risk of atrial fibrillation and clot formation

⇧ risk of stroke (see map)

until decompensation occurs (see CHF map) → pressure from left ventricle travels back to left atrium

to pulmonary veins and capillaries

⇧ preload stretches myocytes

left ventricular remodeling characterized by new sarcomeres laid down in series with old sarcomeres

⇧ pulmonary capillary hydrostatic pressure relative to plasma oncotic pressure

⇧ venous return when patient is supine

• **orthopnea**
• **paroxysmal nocturnal dyspnea**
• **nocturia**

eccentric hypertrophy

heart can become dilated = **dilated cardiomyopathy**

fluid extravasates into interstitial space of lung parenchyma

⇧ risk of **mitral regurgitation** (see map)

pulmonary edema → ⇧ work of breathing

chest x-ray shows:
• Kerley B lines
• peribronchial cuffing
• fluid in fissures
• pleural effusion

rales

dyspnea on exertion

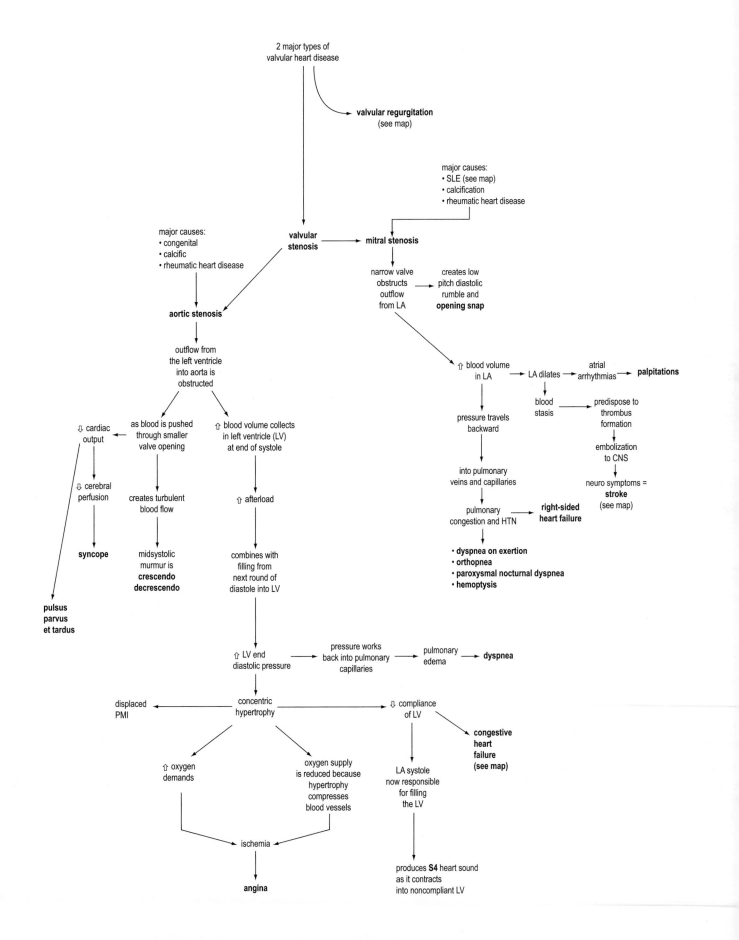

2 major types of
valvular heart disease

valvular regurgitation
(see map)

major causes:
• SLE (see map)
• calcification
• rheumatic heart disease

major causes:
• congenital
• calcific
• rheumatic heart disease

**valvular
stenosis**

mitral stenosis

narrow valve
obstructs
outflow
from LA

creates low
pitch diastolic
rumble and
opening snap

aortic stenosis

outflow from
the left ventricle
into aorta is
obstructed

⇑ blood volume
in LA

LA dilates

atrial
arrhythmias

palpitations

blood
stasis

predispose to
thrombus
formation

pressure travels
backward

embolization
to CNS

⇓ cardiac
output

as blood is pushed
through smaller
valve opening

⇑ blood volume collects
in left ventricle (LV)
at end of systole

into pulmonary
veins and capillaries

neuro symptoms =
stroke
(see map)

⇓ cerebral
perfusion

creates turbulent
blood flow

⇑ afterload

pulmonary
congestion and HTN

**right-sided
heart failure**

syncope

midsystolic
murmur is
**crescendo
decrescendo**

combines with
filling from
next round of
diastole into LV

• **dyspnea on exertion**
• **orthopnea**
• **paroxysmal nocturnal dyspnea**
• **hemoptysis**

**pulsus
parvus
et tardus**

⇑ LV end
diastolic pressure

pressure works
back into pulmonary
capillaries

pulmonary
edema

dyspnea

displaced
PMI

concentric
hypertrophy

⇓ compliance
of LV

**congestive
heart
failure
(see map)**

⇑ oxygen
demands

oxygen supply
is reduced because
hypertrophy
compresses
blood vessels

LA systole
now responsible
for filling
the LV

ischemia

produces **S4** heart sound
as it contracts
into noncompliant LV

angina

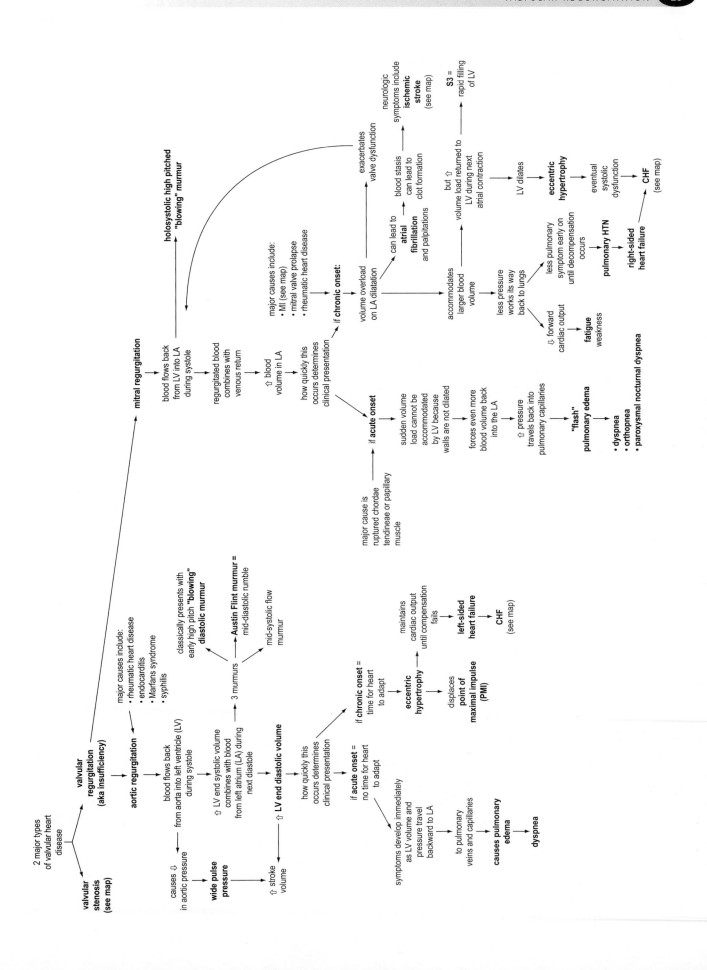

2 major types
of valvular heart
disease

**valvular
stenosis
(see map)**

**valvular
regurgitation
(aka insufficiency)**

aortic regurgitation

causes ⇩
in aortic pressure

**wide pulse
pressure**

⇧ stroke
volume

blood flows back
from aorta into left ventricle (LV)
during systole

⇧ LV end systolic volume
combines with blood
from left atrium (LA) during
next diastole

⇧ LV end diastolic volume

major causes include:
• rheumatic heart disease
• endocarditis
• Marfans syndrome
• syphilis

classically presents with
early high pitch **"blowing"
diastolic murmur**

Austin Flint murmur =
mid-diastolic rumble

3 murmurs

mid-systolic flow
murmur

how quickly this
occurs determines
clinical presentation

if **acute onset** =
no time for heart
to adapt

if **chronic onset** =
time for heart
to adapt

**eccentric
hypertrophy**

maintains
cardiac output
until compensation
fails

**left-sided
heart failure**

CHF
(see map)

displaces
**point of
maximal impulse
(PMI)**

symptoms develop immediately
as LV volume and
pressure travel
backward to LA

to pulmonary
veins and capillaries

**causes pulmonary
edema**

dyspnea

mitral regurgitation

**holosystolic high pitched
"blowing" murmur**

blood flows back
from LV into LA
during systole

regurgitated blood
combines with
venous return

⇧ blood
volume in LA

how quickly this
occurs determines
clinical presentation

major causes include:
• MI (see map)
• mitral valve prolapse
• rheumatic heart disease

if **chronic onset:**

volume overload
on LA dilatation

exacerbates
valve dysfunction

can lead to
**atrial
fibrillation**
and palpitations

blood stasis
can lead to
clot formation

neurologic
symptoms include
**ischemic
stroke**
(see map)

accommodates
larger blood
volume

but ⇧
volume load returned to
LV during next
atrial contraction

S3 =
rapid filling
of LV

LV dilates

**eccentric
hypertrophy**

eventual
systolic
dysfunction

CHF
(see map)

less pressure
works its way
back to lungs

less pulmonary
symptom early on
until decompensation
occurs

pulmonary HTN

**right-sided
heart failure**

⇩ forward
cardiac output

fatigue
weakness

if **acute onset**

major cause is
ruptured chordae
tendineae or papillary
muscle

sudden volume
load cannot be
accommodated
by LV because
walls are not dilated

forces even more
blood volume back
into the LA

⇧ pressure
travels back into
pulmonary capillaries

**"flash"
pulmonary edema**

• **dyspnea**
• **orthopnea**
• **paroxysmal nocturnal dyspnea**

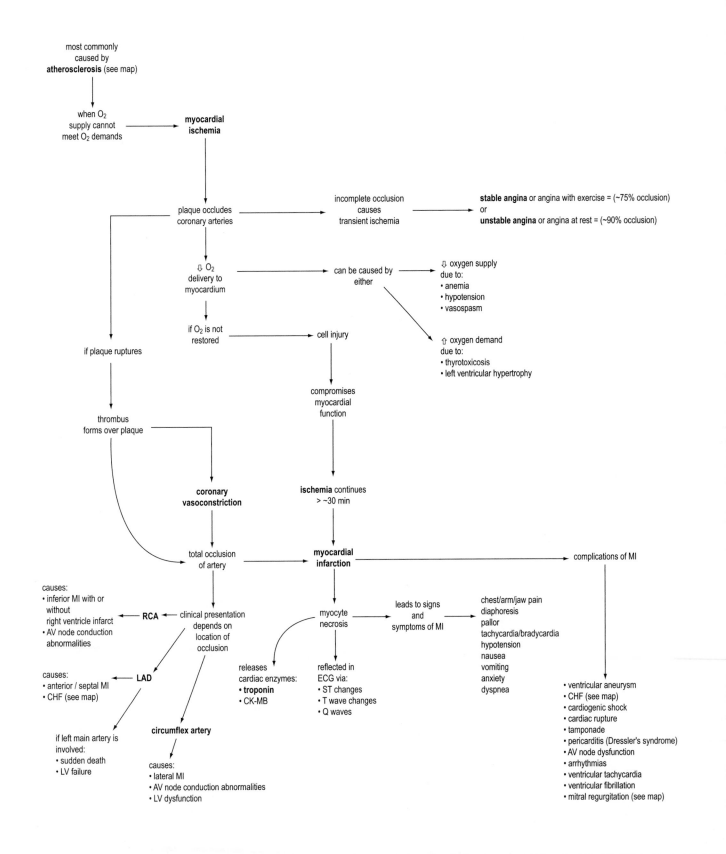

most commonly
caused by
atherosclerosis (see map)

when O₂
supply cannot → **myocardial
meet O₂ demands** **ischemia**

plaque occludes → incomplete occlusion → **stable angina** or angina with exercise = (~75% occlusion)
coronary arteries   causes   or
                      transient ischemia   **unstable angina** or angina at rest = (~90% occlusion)

⇩ O₂ → can be caused by → ⇩ oxygen supply
delivery to   either   due to:
myocardium   • anemia
                            • hypotension
                            • vasospasm

if O₂ is not → cell injury → ⇧ oxygen demand
restored   due to:
                             • thyrotoxicosis
if plaque ruptures   • left ventricular hypertrophy

                compromises
                myocardial
                function

thrombus
forms over plaque

coronary   **ischemia** continues
vasoconstriction   > ~30 min

total occlusion → **myocardial** ──────────────→ complications of MI
of artery   **infarction**

causes: myocyte → leads to signs → chest/arm/jaw pain
• inferior MI with or   necrosis   and   diaphoresis
  without   symptoms of MI pallor
  right ventricle infarct **RCA** ← clinical presentation   tachycardia/bradycardia
• AV node conduction   depends on   hypotension
  abnormalities   location of   nausea
                                 occlusion   vomiting
                                                                         anxiety
causes: **LAD**   releases   reflected in   dyspnea
• anterior / septal MI   cardiac enzymes: ECG via:
• CHF (see map)   • **troponin**   • ST changes   • ventricular aneurysm
                                 • CK-MB   • T wave changes   • CHF (see map)
                                                   • Q waves   • cardiogenic shock
if left main artery is   • cardiac rupture
involved: **circumflex artery**   • tamponade
• sudden death   • pericarditis (Dressler's syndrome)
• LV failure   • AV node dysfunction
                  causes: • arrhythmias
                  • lateral MI   • ventricular tachycardia
                  • AV node conduction abnormalities   • ventricular fibrillation
                  • LV dysfunction   • mitral regurgitation (see map)

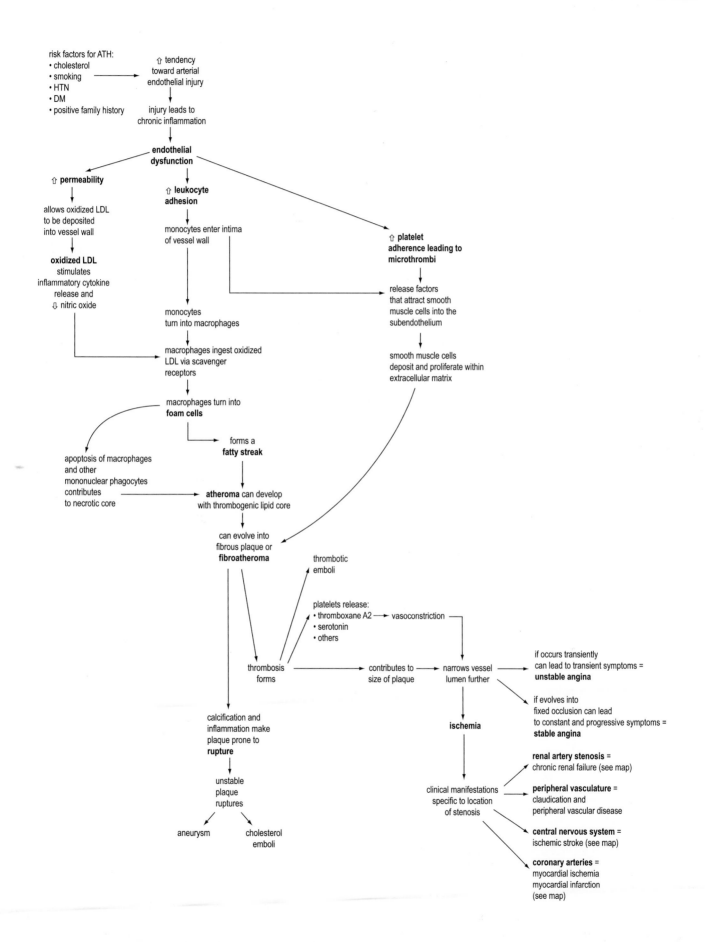

risk factors for ATH:
• cholesterol
• smoking
• HTN
• DM
• positive family history

⇧ tendency toward arterial endothelial injury

injury leads to chronic inflammation

endothelial dysfunction

⇧ **permeability**

allows oxidized LDL to be deposited into vessel wall

oxidized LDL stimulates inflammatory cytokine release and ⇩ nitric oxide

⇧ **leukocyte adhesion**

monocytes enter intima of vessel wall

monocytes turn into macrophages

macrophages ingest oxidized LDL via scavenger receptors

macrophages turn into **foam cells**

⇧ **platelet adherence leading to microthrombi**

release factors that attract smooth muscle cells into the subendothelium

smooth muscle cells deposit and proliferate within extracellular matrix

apoptosis of macrophages and other mononuclear phagocytes contributes to necrotic core

forms a **fatty streak**

atheroma can develop with thrombogenic lipid core

can evolve into fibrous plaque or **fibroatheroma**

thrombotic emboli

platelets release:
• thromboxane A2 ⟶ vasoconstriction
• serotonin
• others

thrombosis forms

contributes to size of plaque

narrows vessel lumen further

if occurs transiently can lead to transient symptoms = **unstable angina**

if evolves into fixed occlusion can lead to constant and progressive symptoms = **stable angina**

ischemia

calcification and inflammation make plaque prone to **rupture**

unstable plaque ruptures

aneurysm

cholesterol emboli

clinical manifestations specific to location of stenosis

renal artery stenosis = chronic renal failure (see map)

peripheral vasculature = claudication and peripheral vascular disease

central nervous system = ischemic stroke (see map)

coronary arteries = myocardial ischemia myocardial infarction (see map)

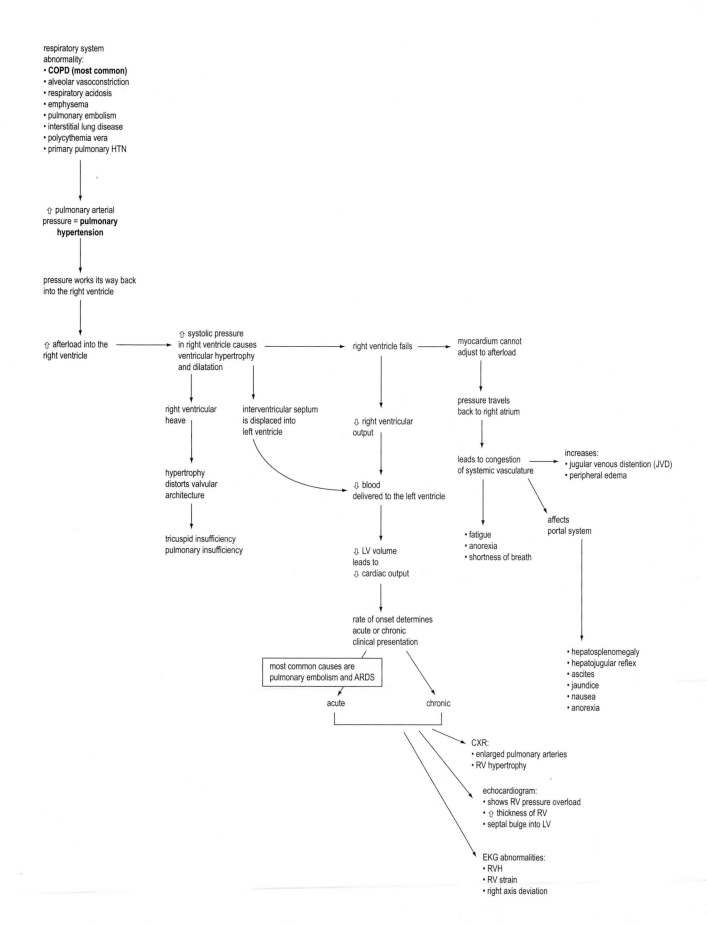

respiratory system
abnormality:
• **COPD (most common)**
• alveolar vasoconstriction
• respiratory acidosis
• emphysema
• pulmonary embolism
• interstitial lung disease
• polycythemia vera
• primary pulmonary HTN

⇧ pulmonary arterial
pressure = **pulmonary
hypertension**

pressure works its way back
into the right ventricle

⇧ afterload into the
right ventricle

⇧ systolic pressure
in right ventricle causes
ventricular hypertrophy
and dilatation

right ventricle fails

myocardium cannot
adjust to afterload

right ventricular
heave

interventricular septum
is displaced into
left ventricle

⇩ right ventricular
output

pressure travels
back to right atrium

hypertrophy
distorts valvular
architecture

⇩ blood
delivered to the left ventricle

leads to congestion
of systemic vasculature

increases:
• jugular venous distention (JVD)
• peripheral edema

tricuspid insufficiency
pulmonary insufficiency

⇩ LV volume
leads to
⇩ cardiac output

• fatigue
• anorexia
• shortness of breath

affects
portal system

rate of onset determines
acute or chronic
clinical presentation

• hepatosplenomegaly
• hepatojugular reflex
• ascites
• jaundice
• nausea
• anorexia

most common causes are
pulmonary embolism and ARDS

acute   chronic

CXR:
• enlarged pulmonary arteries
• RV hypertrophy

echocardiogram:
• shows RV pressure overload
• ⇧ thickness of RV
• septal bulge into LV

EKG abnormalities:
• RVH
• RV strain
• right axis deviation

Pulmonary Disorders

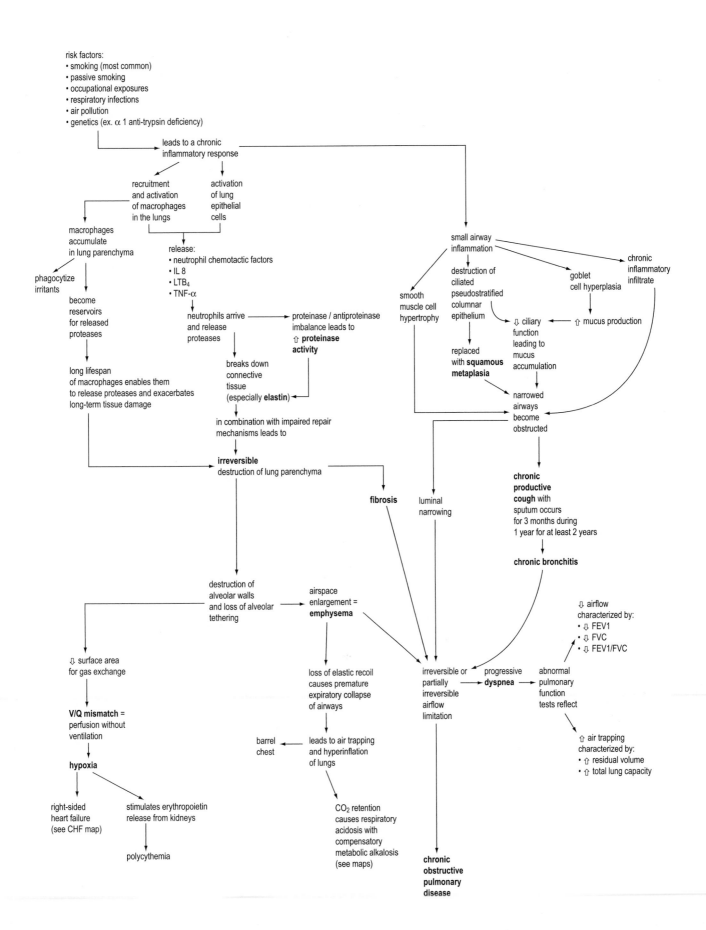

risk factors:
• smoking (most common)
• passive smoking
• occupational exposures
• respiratory infections
• air pollution
• genetics (ex. α 1 anti-trypsin deficiency)

leads to a chronic inflammatory response

recruitment and activation of macrophages in the lungs

activation of lung epithelial cells

macrophages accumulate in lung parenchyma

phagocytize irritants

become reservoirs for released proteases

long lifespan of macrophages enables them to release proteases and exacerbates long-term tissue damage

release:
• neutrophil chemotactic factors
• IL 8
• LTB_4
• TNF-α

neutrophils arrive and release proteases

proteinase / antiproteinase imbalance leads to ⇧ **proteinase activity**

breaks down connective tissue (especially **elastin**)

in combination with impaired repair mechanisms leads to

irreversible destruction of lung parenchyma

small airway inflammation

smooth muscle cell hypertrophy

destruction of ciliated pseudostratified columnar epithelium

goblet cell hyperplasia

chronic inflammatory infiltrate

⇩ ciliary function leading to mucus accumulation

⇧ mucus production

replaced with **squamous metaplasia**

narrowed airways become obstructed

fibrosis

luminal narrowing

chronic productive cough with sputum occurs for 3 months during 1 year for at least 2 years

chronic bronchitis

destruction of alveolar walls and loss of alveolar tethering

airspace enlargement = **emphysema**

⇩ surface area for gas exchange

V/Q mismatch = perfusion without ventilation

hypoxia

right-sided heart failure (see CHF map)

stimulates erythropoietin release from kidneys

polycythemia

loss of elastic recoil causes premature expiratory collapse of airways

barrel chest

leads to air trapping and hyperinflation of lungs

CO_2 retention causes respiratory acidosis with compensatory metabolic alkalosis (see maps)

irreversible or partially irreversible airflow limitation

progressive **dyspnea**

abnormal pulmonary function tests reflect

⇩ airflow characterized by:
• ⇩ FEV1
• ⇩ FVC
• ⇩ FEV1/FVC

⇧ air trapping characterized by:
• ⇧ residual volume
• ⇧ total lung capacity

chronic obstructive pulmonary disease

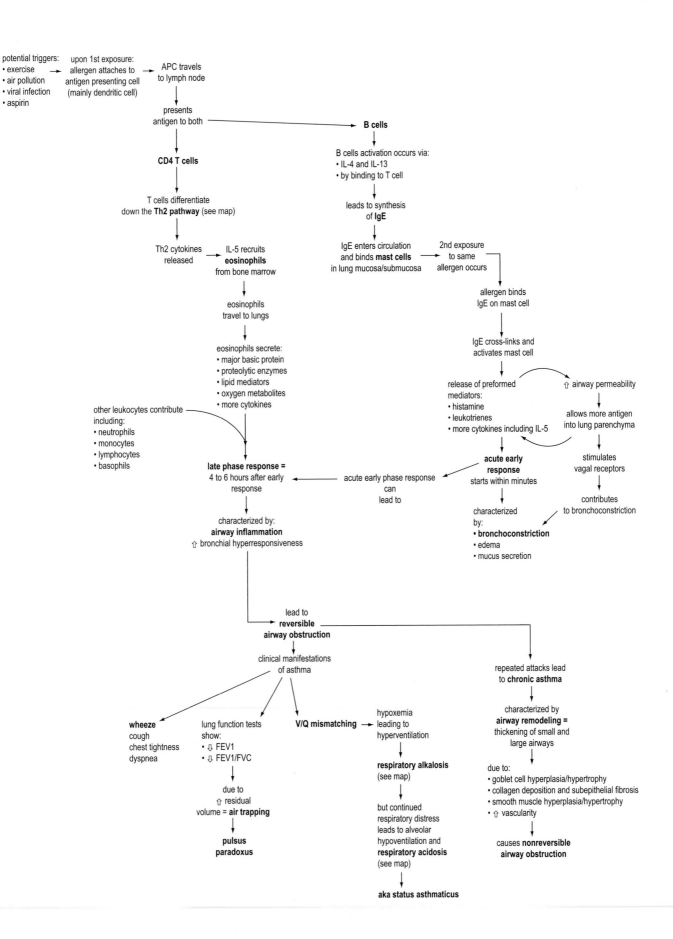

potential triggers:
• exercise
• air pollution
• viral infection
• aspirin

upon 1st exposure:
allergen attaches to
antigen presenting cell
(mainly dendritic cell)

APC travels
to lymph node

presents
antigen to both

B cells

CD4 T cells

B cells activation occurs via:
• IL-4 and IL-13
• by binding to T cell

T cells differentiate
down the **Th2 pathway** (see map)

leads to synthesis
of **IgE**

Th2 cytokines
released

IL-5 recruits
eosinophils
from bone marrow

IgE enters circulation
and binds **mast cells**
in lung mucosa/submucosa

2nd exposure
to same
allergen occurs

allergen binds
IgE on mast cell

eosinophils
travel to lungs

IgE cross-links and
activates mast cell

eosinophils secrete:
• major basic protein
• proteolytic enzymes
• lipid mediators
• oxygen metabolites
• more cytokines

release of preformed
mediators:
• histamine
• leukotrienes
• more cytokines including IL-5

⇑ airway permeability

allows more antigen
into lung parenchyma

other leukocytes contribute
including:
• neutrophils
• monocytes
• lymphocytes
• basophils

**acute early
response**
starts within minutes

stimulates
vagal receptors

late phase response =
4 to 6 hours after early
response

acute early phase response
can
lead to

characterized
by:
• **bronchoconstriction**
• edema
• mucus secretion

contributes
to bronchoconstriction

characterized by:
airway inflammation
⇑ bronchial hyperresponsiveness

lead to
**reversible
airway obstruction**

clinical manifestations
of asthma

repeated attacks lead
to **chronic asthma**

wheeze
cough
chest tightness
dyspnea

lung function tests
show:
• ⇓ FEV1
• ⇓ FEV1/FVC

V/Q mismatching

hypoxemia
leading to
hyperventilation

characterized by
airway remodeling =
thickening of small and
large airways

respiratory alkalosis
(see map)

due to:
• goblet cell hyperplasia/hypertrophy
• collagen deposition and subepithelial fibrosis
• smooth muscle hyperplasia/hypertrophy
• ⇑ vascularity

due to
⇑ residual
volume = **air trapping**

but continued
respiratory distress
leads to alveolar
hypoventilation and
respiratory acidosis
(see map)

causes **nonreversible
airway obstruction**

**pulsus
paradoxus**

aka status asthmaticus

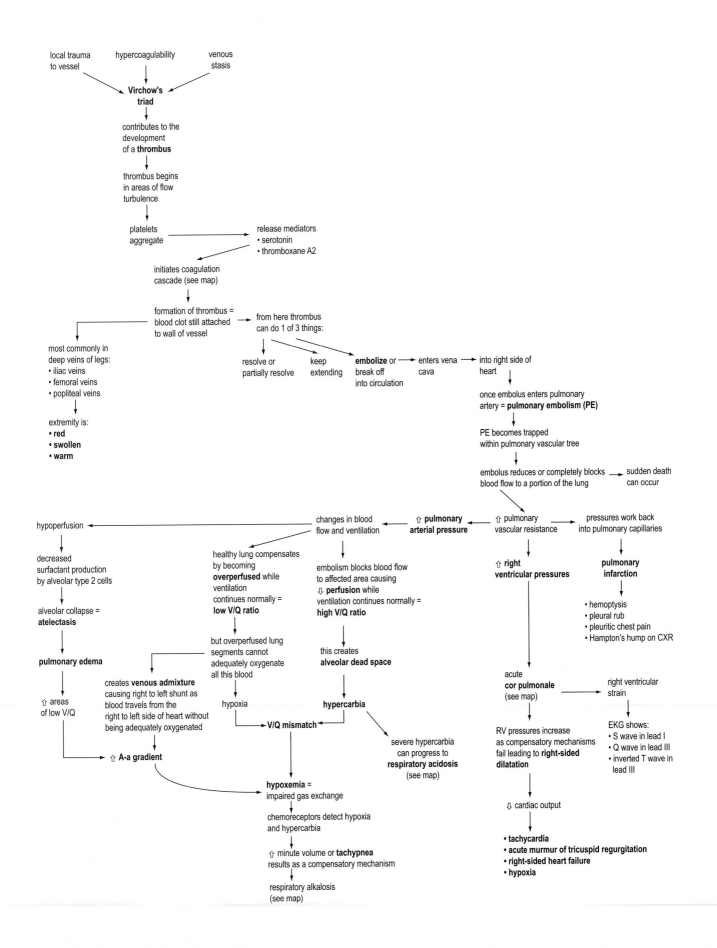

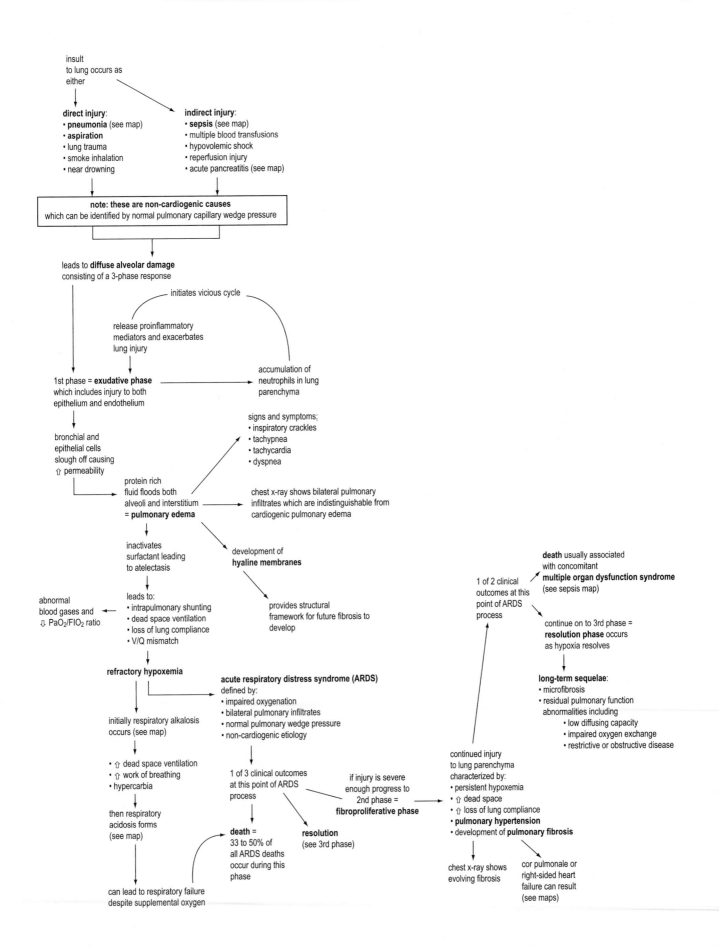

insult
to lung occurs as
either

direct injury:
• **pneumonia** (see map)
• **aspiration**
• lung trauma
• smoke inhalation
• near drowning

indirect injury:
• **sepsis** (see map)
• multiple blood transfusions
• hypovolemic shock
• reperfusion injury
• acute pancreatitis (see map)

note: these are non-cardiogenic causes
which can be identified by normal pulmonary capillary wedge pressure

leads to **diffuse alveolar damage**
consisting of a 3-phase response

initiates vicious cycle

release proinflammatory
mediators and exacerbates
lung injury

accumulation of
neutrophils in lung
parenchyma

1st phase = **exudative phase**
which includes injury to both
epithelium and endothelium

bronchial and
epithelial cells
slough off causing
⇧ permeability

signs and symptoms;
• inspiratory crackles
• tachypnea
• tachycardia
• dyspnea

protein rich
fluid floods both
alveoli and interstitium
= **pulmonary edema**

chest x-ray shows bilateral pulmonary
infiltrates which are indistinguishable from
cardiogenic pulmonary edema

inactivates
surfactant leading
to atelectasis

development of
hyaline membranes

abnormal
blood gases and
⇩ PaO_2/FIO_2 ratio

leads to:
• intrapulmonary shunting
• dead space ventilation
• loss of lung compliance
• V/Q mismatch

provides structural
framework for future fibrosis to
develop

refractory hypoxemia

acute respiratory distress syndrome (ARDS)
defined by:
• impaired oxygenation
• bilateral pulmonary infiltrates
• normal pulmonary wedge pressure
• non-cardiogenic etiology

initially respiratory alkalosis
occurs (see map)

• ⇧ dead space ventilation
• ⇧ work of breathing
• hypercarbia

then respiratory
acidosis forms
(see map)

1 of 3 clinical outcomes
at this point of ARDS
process

if injury is severe
enough progress to
2nd phase =
fibroproliferative phase

death =
33 to 50% of
all ARDS deaths
occur during this
phase

resolution
(see 3rd phase)

can lead to respiratory failure
despite supplemental oxygen

continued injury
to lung parenchyma
characterized by:
• persistent hypoxemia
• ⇧ dead space
• ⇧ loss of lung compliance
• **pulmonary hypertension**
• development of **pulmonary fibrosis**

chest x-ray shows
evolving fibrosis

cor pulmonale or
right-sided heart
failure can result
(see maps)

1 of 2 clinical
outcomes at this
point of ARDS
process

death usually associated
with concomitant
multiple organ dysfunction syndrome
(see sepsis map)

continue on to 3rd phase =
resolution phase occurs
as hypoxia resolves

long-term sequelae:
• microfibrosis
• residual pulmonary function
abnormalities including
     • low diffusing capacity
     • impaired oxygen exchange
     • restrictive or obstructive disease

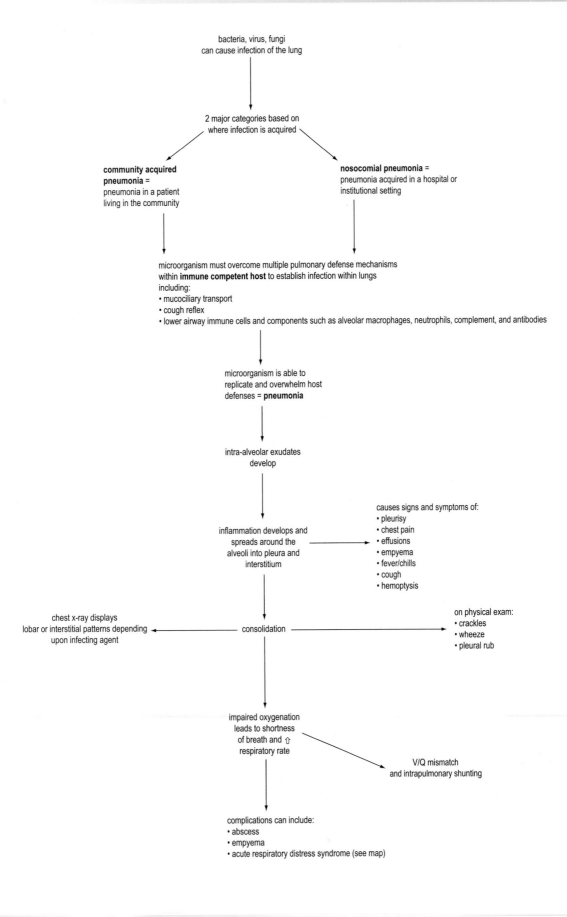

bacteria, virus, fungi
can cause infection of the lung

2 major categories based on
where infection is acquired

**community acquired
pneumonia** =
pneumonia in a patient
living in the community

nosocomial pneumonia =
pneumonia acquired in a hospital or
institutional setting

microorganism must overcome multiple pulmonary defense mechanisms
within **immune competent host** to establish infection within lungs
including:
• mucociliary transport
• cough reflex
• lower airway immune cells and components such as alveolar macrophages, neutrophils, complement, and antibodies

microorganism is able to
replicate and overwhelm host
defenses = **pneumonia**

intra-alveolar exudates
develop

inflammation develops and
spreads around the
alveoli into pleura and
interstitium

causes signs and symptoms of:
• pleurisy
• chest pain
• effusions
• empyema
• fever/chills
• cough
• hemoptysis

chest x-ray displays
lobar or interstitial patterns depending
upon infecting agent

consolidation

on physical exam:
• crackles
• wheeze
• pleural rub

impaired oxygenation
leads to shortness
of breath and ⇧
respiratory rate

V/Q mismatch
and intrapulmonary shunting

complications can include:
• abscess
• empyema
• acute respiratory distress syndrome (see map)

Genetic Disorders

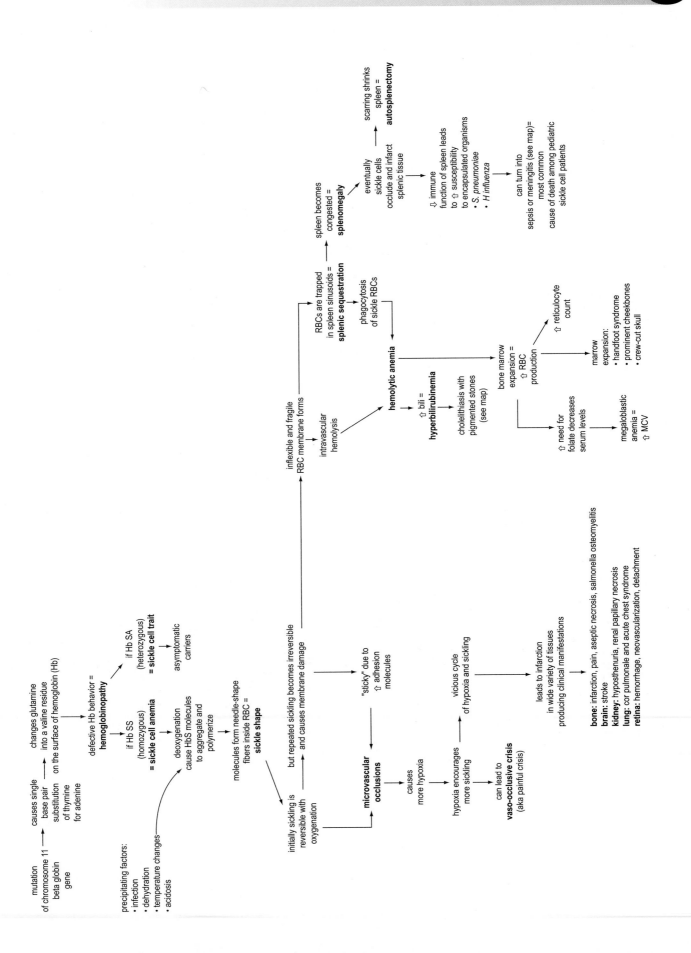

mutation
of chromosome 11 → causes single → base pair substitution → changes glutamine into a valine residue
beta globin gene   of thymine for adenine   on the surface of hemoglobin (Hb)

defective Hb behavior = **hemoglobinopathy**

if Hb SA (heterozygous) = **sickle cell trait** → asymptomatic carriers

if Hb SS (homozygous) = **sickle cell anemia**

precipitating factors:
• infection
• dehydration
• temperature changes
• acidosis

deoxygenation cause HbS molecules to aggregate and polymerize

molecules form needle-shape fibers inside RBC = **sickle shape**

initially sickling is reversible with oxygenation

but repeated sickling becomes irreversible and causes membrane damage

"sticky" due to ⇧ adhesion molecules

microvascular occlusions

causes more hypoxia

hypoxia encourages more sickling

vicious cycle of hypoxia and sickling

can lead to **vaso-occlusive crisis** (aka painful crisis)

leads to infarction in wide variety of tissues producing clinical manifestations

bone: infarction, pain, aseptic necrosis, salmonella osteomyelitis
brain: stroke
kidney: hyposthenuria, renal papillary necrosis
lung: cor pulmonale and acute chest syndrome
retina: hemorrhage, neovascularization, detachment

inflexible and fragile RBC membrane forms

intravascular hemolysis

RBCs are trapped in spleen sinusoids = **splenic sequestration**

phagocytosis of sickle RBCs

hemolytic anemia

⇧ bili = **hyperbilirubinemia** → cholelithiasis with pigmented stones (see map)

bone marrow expansion = ⇧ RBC production

⇧ reticulocyte count

marrow expansion:
• handfoot syndrome
• prominent cheekbones
• crew-cut skull

⇧ need for folate decreases serum levels

megaloblastic anemia = ⇧ MCV

spleen becomes congested = **splenomegaly**

eventually sickle cells occlude and infarct splenic tissue

scarring shrinks spleen = **autosplenectomy**

⇩ immune function of spleen leads to ⇧ susceptibility to encapsulated organisms
• *S. pneumoniae*
• *H influenza*

can turn into sepsis or meningitis (see map) = most common cause of death among pediatric sickle cell patients

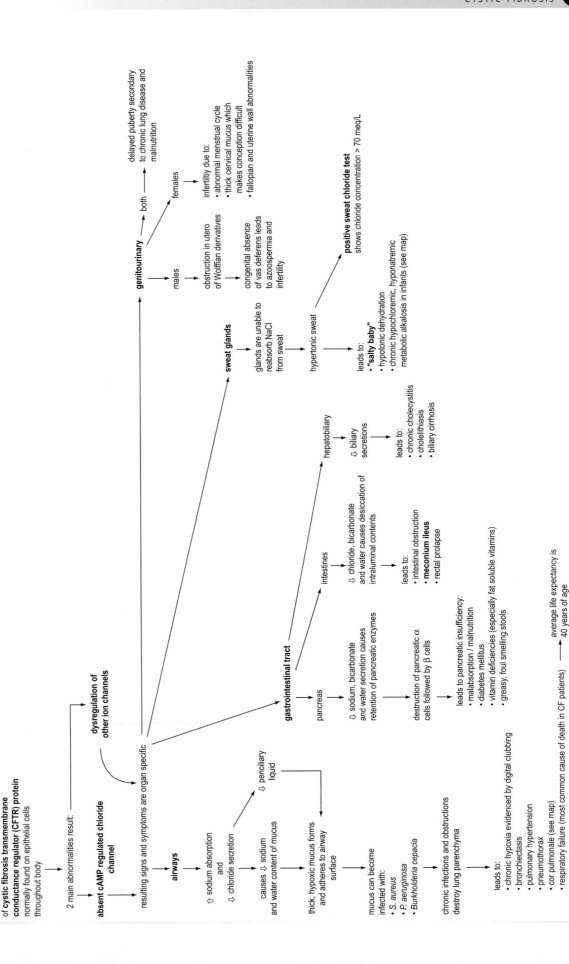

multiple autosomal recessive
genetic mutations possible
but most common type is **delta F508**

disrupts production
of **cystic fibrosis transmembrane
conductance regulator (CFTR) protein**
normally found on epithelial cells
throughout body

2 main abnormalities result:

**absent cAMP regulated chloride
channel**

**dysregulation of
other ion channels**

resulting signs and symptoms are organ specific

airways

⇧ sodium absorption
and
⇩ chloride secretion

⇩ periciliary
liquid

causes ⇩ sodium
and water content of mucus

thick, hypoxic mucus forms
and adheres to airway
surface

mucus can become
infected with:
• *S. aureus*
• *P. aeruginosa*
• *Burkholderia cepacia*

chronic infections and obstructions
destroy lung parenchyma

leads to:
• chronic hypoxia evidenced by digital clubbing
• bronchiectasis
• pulmonary hypertension
• pneumothorax
• cor pulmonale (see map)
• respiratory failure (most common cause of death in CF patients) → average life expectancy is
40 years of age

gastrointestinal tract

pancreas

⇩ sodium, bicarbonate
and water secretion causes
retention of pancreatic enzymes

destruction of pancreatic α
cells followed by β cells

leads to pancreatic insufficiency:
• malabsorption / malnutrition
• diabetes mellitus
• vitamin deficiencies (especially fat soluble vitamins)
• greasy, foul smelling stools

intestines

⇩ chloride, bicarbonate
and water causes desiccation of
intraluminal contents

leads to:
• intestinal obstruction
• **meconium ileus**
• rectal prolapse

hepatobiliary

⇩ biliary
secretions

leads to:
• chronic cholecystitis
• cholelithiasis
• biliary cirrhosis

sweat glands

glands are unable to
reabsorb NaCl
from sweat

hypertonic sweat

leads to:
• **"salty baby"**
• hypotonic dehydration
• chronic hypochloremic, hyponatremic
metabolic alkalosis in infants (see map)

positive sweat chloride test
shows chloride concentration > 70 meq/L

genitourinary → both → delayed puberty secondary
to chronic lung disease and
malnutrition

females

infertility due to:
• abnormal menstrual cycle
• thick cervical mucus which
makes conception difficult
• fallopian and uterine wall abnormalities

males

obstruction in utero
of Wolffian derivatives

congenital absence
of vas deferens leads
to azoospermia and
infertility

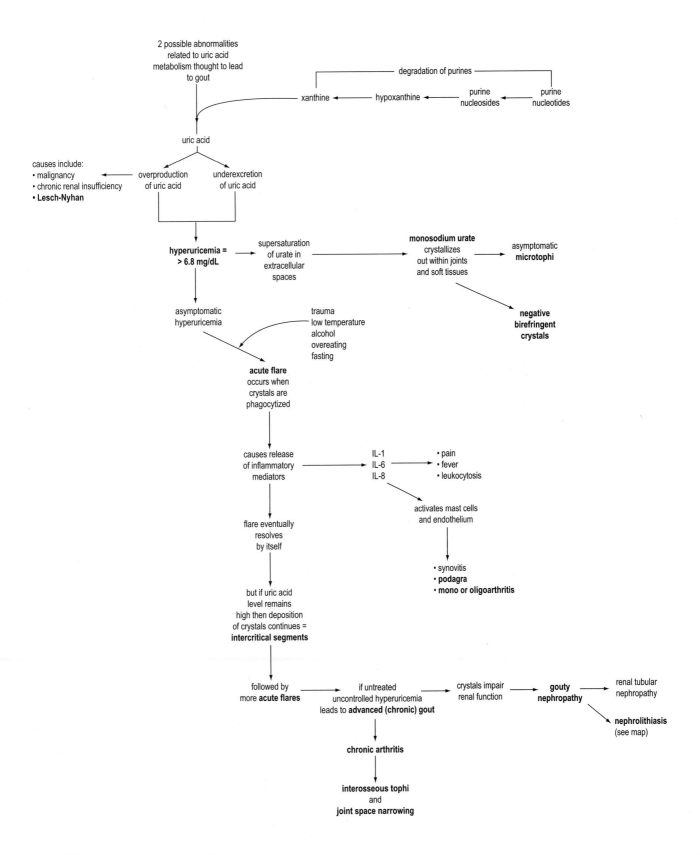

2 possible abnormalities
related to uric acid
metabolism thought to lead
to gout

degradation of purines

xanthine ← hypoxanthine ← purine
nucleosides ← purine
nucleotides

uric acid

causes include:
• malignancy
• chronic renal insufficiency
• **Lesch-Nyhan**

overproduction
of uric acid ← → underexcretion
of uric acid

**hyperuricemia =
> 6.8 mg/dL**

supersaturation
of urate in
extracellular
spaces

monosodium urate
crystallizes
out within joints
and soft tissues

asymptomatic
microtophi

**negative
birefringent
crystals**

asymptomatic
hyperuricemia

trauma
low temperature
alcohol
overeating
fasting

acute flare
occurs when
crystals are
phagocytized

causes release
of inflammatory
mediators

IL-1
IL-6
IL-8

• pain
• fever
• leukocytosis

activates mast cells
and endothelium

flare eventually
resolves
by itself

• synovitis
• **podagra**
• **mono or oligoarthritis**

but if uric acid
level remains
high then deposition
of crystals continues =
intercritical segments

followed by
more **acute flares**

if untreated
uncontrolled hyperuricemia
leads to **advanced (chronic) gout**

crystals impair
renal function

**gouty
nephropathy**

renal tubular
nephropathy

nephrolithiasis
(see map)

chronic arthritis

interosseous tophi
and
joint space narrowing

Hemostasis Disorders

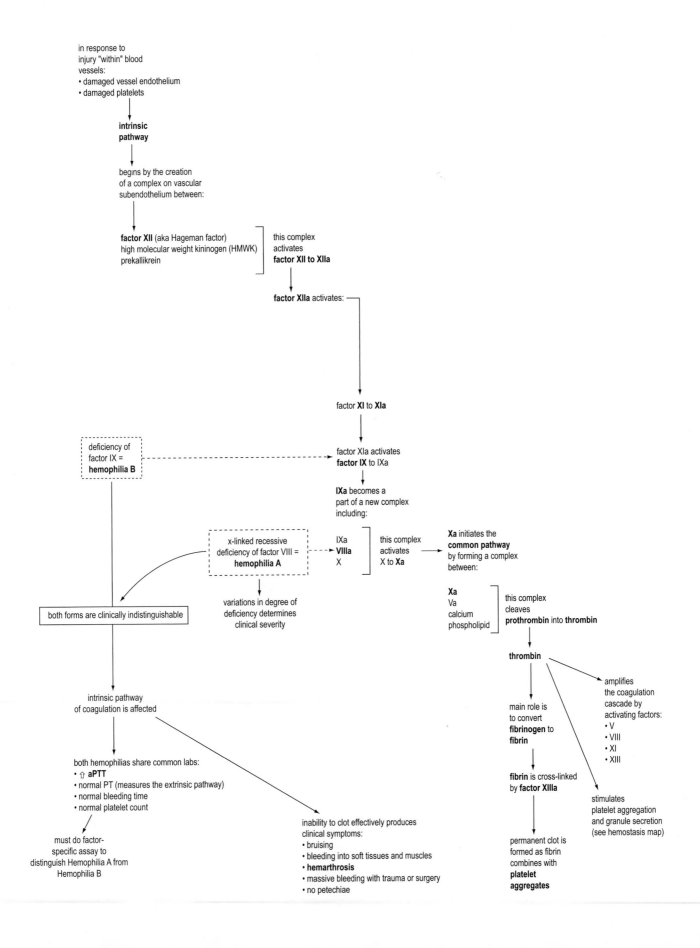

in response to
injury "within" blood
vessels:
• damaged vessel endothelium
• damaged platelets

**intrinsic
pathway**

begins by the creation
of a complex on vascular
subendothelium between:

factor XII (aka Hageman factor)
high molecular weight kininogen (HMWK)
prekallikrein

this complex
activates
factor XII to XIIa

factor XIIa activates:

factor **XI** to **XIa**

deficiency of
factor IX =
hemophilia B

factor XIa activates
factor IX to IXa

IXa becomes a
part of a new complex
including:

x-linked recessive
deficiency of factor VIII =
hemophilia A

IXa
VIIIa
X

this complex
activates
X to **Xa**

Xa initiates the
common pathway
by forming a complex
between:

both forms are clinically indistinguishable

variations in degree of
deficiency determines
clinical severity

Xa
Va
calcium
phospholipid

this complex
cleaves
prothrombin into **thrombin**

thrombin

amplifies
the coagulation
cascade by
activating factors:
• V
• VIII
• XI
• XIII

intrinsic pathway
of coagulation is affected

main role is
to convert
fibrinogen to
fibrin

both hemophilias share common labs:
• ⇧ **aPTT**
• normal PT (measures the extrinsic pathway)
• normal bleeding time
• normal platelet count

fibrin is cross-linked
by **factor XIIIa**

stimulates
platelet aggregation
and granule secretion
(see hemostasis map)

must do factor-
specific assay to
distinguish Hemophilia A from
Hemophilia B

inability to clot effectively produces
clinical symptoms:
• bruising
• bleeding into soft tissues and muscles
• **hemarthrosis**
• massive bleeding with trauma or surgery
• no petechiae

permanent clot is
formed as fibrin
combines with
**platelet
aggregates**

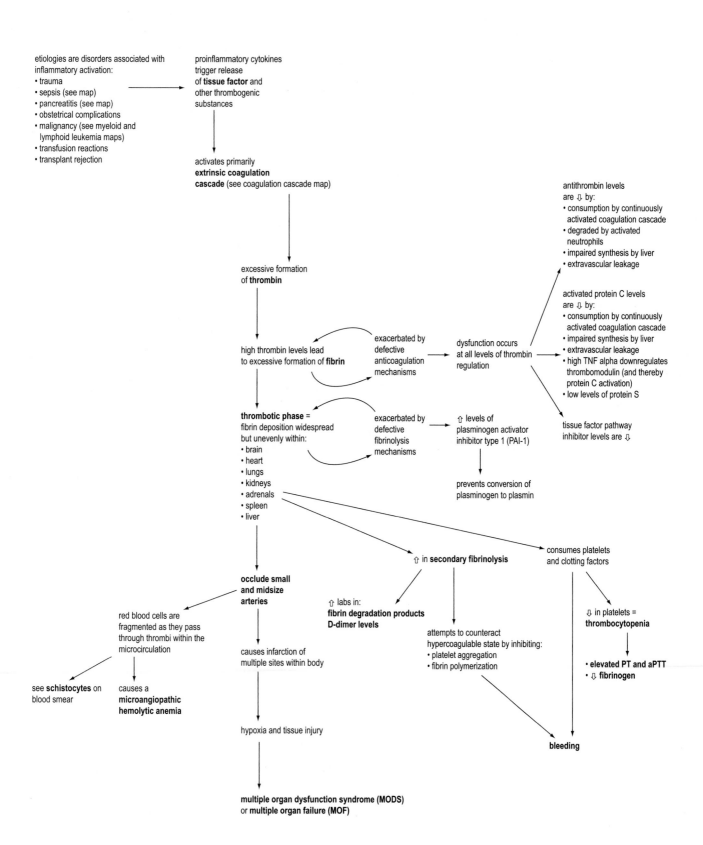

etiologies are disorders associated with inflammatory activation:
• trauma
• sepsis (see map)
• pancreatitis (see map)
• obstetrical complications
• malignancy (see myeloid and lymphoid leukemia maps)
• transfusion reactions
• transplant rejection

proinflammatory cytokines trigger release of **tissue factor** and other thrombogenic substances

activates primarily **extrinsic coagulation cascade** (see coagulation cascade map)

excessive formation of **thrombin**

high thrombin levels lead to excessive formation of **fibrin**

exacerbated by defective anticoagulation mechanisms

dysfunction occurs at all levels of thrombin regulation

antithrombin levels are ⇩ by:
• consumption by continuously activated coagulation cascade
• degraded by activated neutrophils
• impaired synthesis by liver
• extravascular leakage

activated protein C levels are ⇩ by:
• consumption by continuously activated coagulation cascade
• impaired synthesis by liver
• extravascular leakage
• high TNF alpha downregulates thrombomodulin (and thereby protein C activation)
• low levels of protein S

thrombotic phase = fibrin deposition widespread but unevenly within:
• brain
• heart
• lungs
• kidneys
• adrenals
• spleen
• liver

exacerbated by defective fibrinolysis mechanisms

⇧ levels of plasminogen activator inhibitor type 1 (PAI-1)

tissue factor pathway inhibitor levels are ⇩

prevents conversion of plasminogen to plasmin

consumes platelets and clotting factors

⇧ in **secondary fibrinolysis**

occlude small and midsize arteries

red blood cells are fragmented as they pass through thrombi within the microcirculation

⇧ labs in:
fibrin degradation products D-dimer levels

attempts to counteract hypercoagulable state by inhibiting:
• platelet aggregation
• fibrin polymerization

⇩ in platelets = **thrombocytopenia**

• **elevated PT and aPTT**
• ⇩ **fibrinogen**

see **schistocytes** on blood smear

causes a **microangiopathic hemolytic anemia**

causes infarction of multiple sites within body

hypoxia and tissue injury

bleeding

multiple organ dysfunction syndrome (MODS) or **multiple organ failure (MOF)**

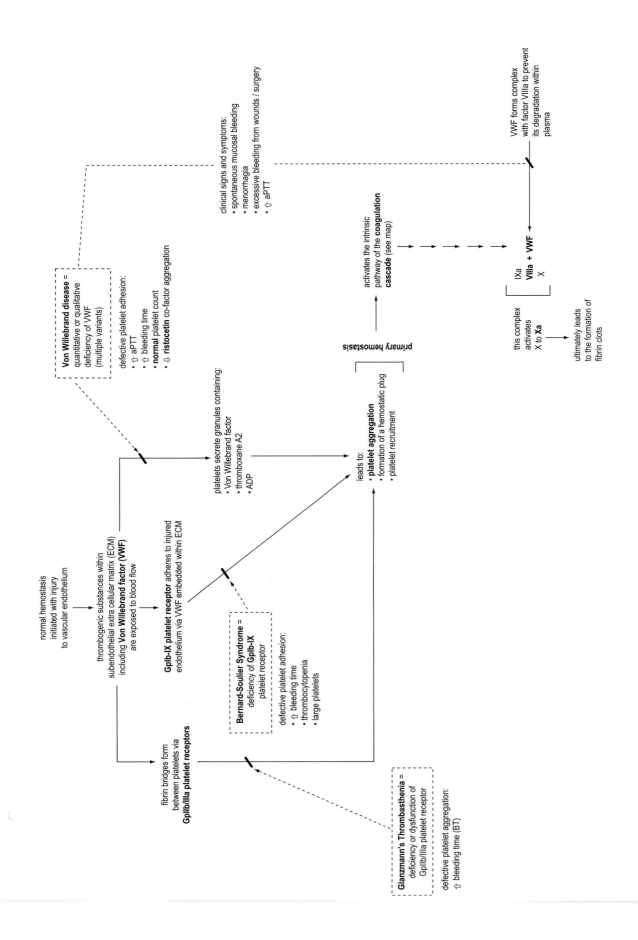

normal hemostasis
initiated with injury
to vascular endothelium

thrombogenic substances within
subendothelial extra cellular matrix (ECM)
including **Von Willebrand factor (VWF)**
are exposed to blood flow

GpIb-IX platelet receptor adheres to injured
endothelium via VWF embedded within ECM

fibrin bridges form
between platelets via
GpIIb/IIIa platelet receptors

Bernard-Soulier Syndrome =
deficiency of **GpIb-IX**
platelet receptor

defective platelet adhesion:
• ⇧ bleeding time
• thrombocytopenia
• large platelets

Glanzmann's Thrombasthenia =
deficiency or dysfunction of
GpIIb/IIIa platelet receptor

defective platelet aggregation:
⇧ bleeding time (BT)

Von Willebrand disease =
quantitative or qualitative
deficiency of VWF
(multiple variants)

defective platelet adhesion:
• ⇧ aPTT
• ⇧ bleeding time
• **normal** platelet count
• ⇩ **ristocetin** co-factor aggregation

platelets secrete granules containing:
• Von Willebrand factor
• thromboxane A2
• ADP

leads to:
• **platelet aggregation**
• formation of a hemostatic plug
• platelet recruitment

primary hemostasis

clinical signs and symptoms:
• spontaneous mucosal bleeding
• menorrhagia
• excessive bleeding from wounds / surgery
• ⇧ aPTT

activates the intrinsic
pathway of the **coagulation
cascade** (see map)

VWF forms complex
with factor VIIIa to prevent
its degradation within
plasma

IXa
VIIIa + VWF
X

this complex
activates
X to **Xa**

ultimately leads
to the formation of
fibrin clots

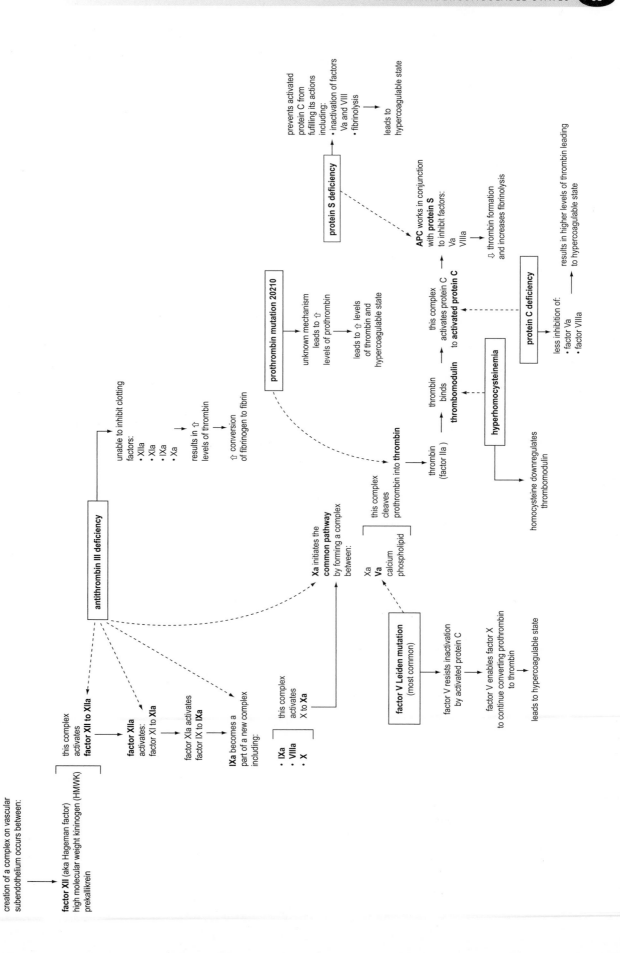

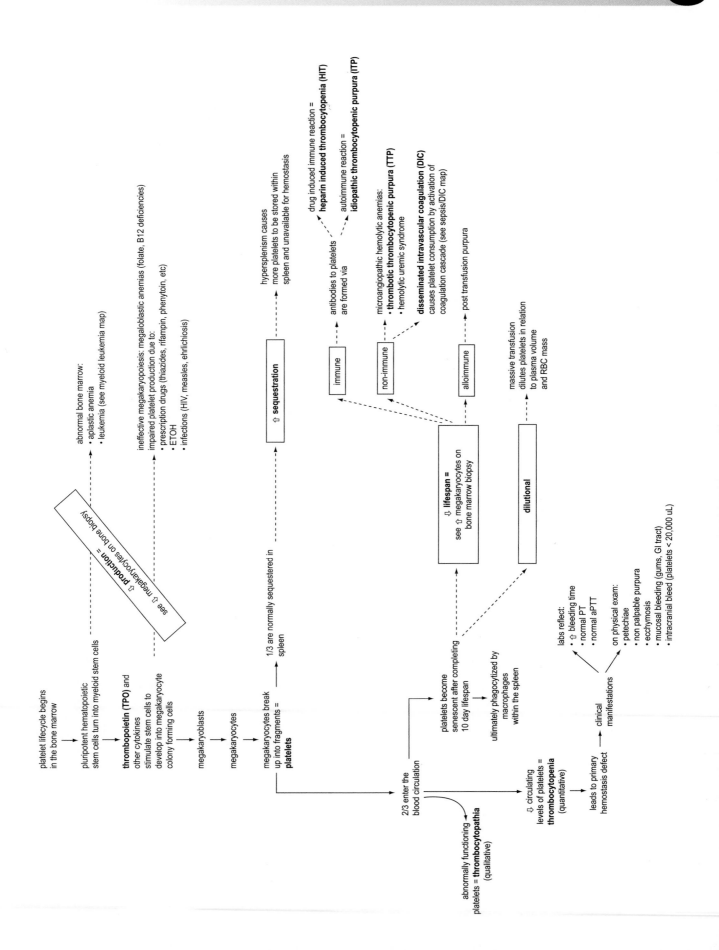

platelet lifecycle begins in the bone marrow

pluripotent hematopoietic stem cells turn into myeloid stem cells

thrombopoietin (TPO) and other cytokines stimulate stem cells to develop into megakaryocyte colony forming cells

megakaryoblasts

megakaryocytes

megakaryocytes break up into fragments = **platelets**

production = see ⇧ megakaryocytes on bone biopsy

abnormal bone marrow:
• aplastic anemia
• leukemia (see myeloid leukemia map)

ineffective megakaryopoiesis: megaloblastic anemias (folate, B12 deficiencies)
impaired platelet production due to:
• prescription drugs (thiazides, rifampin, phenytoin, etc)
• ETOH
• infections (HIV, measles, ehrlichiosis)

1/3 are normally sequestered in spleen

⇧ **sequestration**

hypersplenism causes more platelets to be stored within spleen and unavailable for hemostasis

2/3 enter the blood circulation

⇩ circulating levels of platelets = **thrombocytopenia** (quantitative)

abnormally functioning platelets = **thrombocytopathia** (qualitative)

leads to primary hemostasis defect

platelets become senescent after completing 10 day lifespan

ultimately phagocytized by macrophages within the spleen

⇩ **lifespan** = see ⇧ megakaryocytes on bone marrow biopsy

immune

antibodies to platelets are formed via

drug induced immune reaction = **heparin induced thrombocytopenia (HIT)**

autoimmune reaction = **idiopathic thrombocytopenic purpura (ITP)**

non-immune

microangiopathic hemolytic anemias:
• **thrombotic thrombocytopenic purpura (TTP)**
• hemolytic uremic syndrome

disseminated intravascular coagulation (DIC) causes platelet consumption by activation of coagulation cascade (see sepsis/DIC map)

alloimmune

post transfusion purpura

dilutional

massive transfusion dilutes platelets in relation to plasma volume and RBC mass

clinical manifestations

labs reflect:
• ⇧ bleeding time
• normal PT
• normal aPTT

on physical exam:
• petechiae
• non palpable purpura
• ecchymosis
• mucosal bleeding (gums, GI tract)
• intracranial bleed (platelets < 20,000 uL)

Hematopoietic Disorders

Hemoglobin A (adult hemoglobin) is composed of:
• **2 α chains**
• 2 β chains

→ **α globin chains** are produced under the direction of 4 α globin genes

→ genetic mutations result in abnormal α globin chain synthesis

defective hemoglobin synthesis causing a hypochromic anemia = **alpha thalassemia**

mutations can affect between 1 to all 4 α globin genes

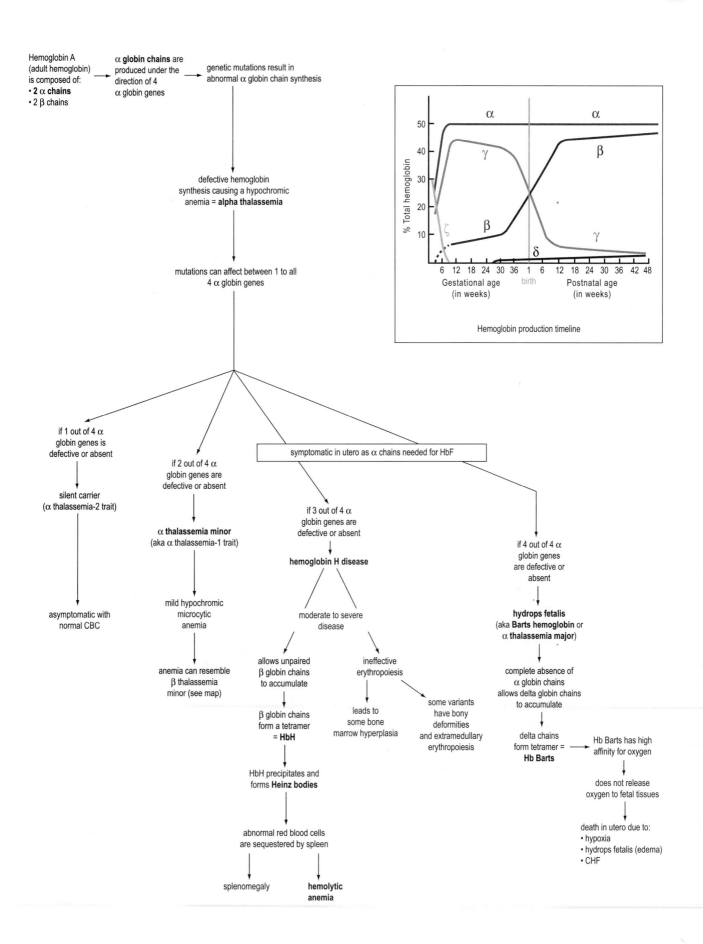

Hemoglobin production timeline

if 1 out of 4 α globin genes is defective or absent

silent carrier (α thalassemia-2 trait)

asymptomatic with normal CBC

if 2 out of 4 α globin genes are defective or absent

α thalassemia minor (aka α thalassemia-1 trait)

mild hypochromic microcytic anemia

anemia can resemble β thalassemia minor (see map)

symptomatic in utero as α chains needed for HbF

if 3 out of 4 α globin genes are defective or absent

hemoglobin H disease

moderate to severe disease

allows unpaired β globin chains to accumulate

β globin chains form a tetramer = **HbH**

HbH precipitates and forms **Heinz bodies**

abnormal red blood cells are sequestered by spleen

splenomegaly

hemolytic anemia

ineffective erythropoiesis

leads to some bone marrow hyperplasia

some variants have bony deformities and extramedullary erythropoiesis

if 4 out of 4 α globin genes are defective or absent

hydrops fetalis (aka **Barts hemoglobin** or α **thalassemia major**)

complete absence of α globin chains allows delta globin chains to accumulate

delta chains form tetramer = **Hb Barts**

Hb Barts has high affinity for oxygen

does not release oxygen to fetal tissues

death in utero due to:
• hypoxia
• hydrops fetalis (edema)
• CHF

Hemoglobin A (adult hemoglobin) is composed of:
• 2 α chains
• **2 β chains**

→ **β globin chains** are produced under the direction of 2 β globin genes

→ defective β globin chain production causes a hypochromic anemia = **β thalassemia**

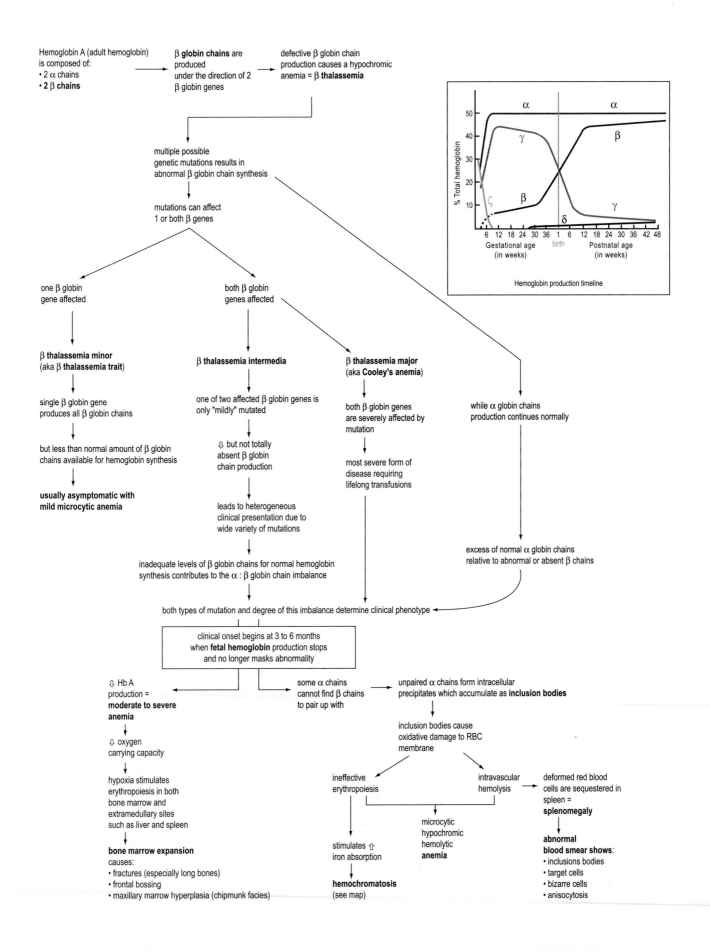

Hemoglobin production timeline

multiple possible genetic mutations results in abnormal β globin chain synthesis

mutations can affect 1 or both β genes

one β globin gene affected

both β globin genes affected

β thalassemia minor (aka β **thalassemia trait**)

single β globin gene produces all β globin chains

but less than normal amount of β globin chains available for hemoglobin synthesis

usually asymptomatic with mild microcytic anemia

β thalassemia intermedia

one of two affected β globin genes is only "mildly" mutated

⇩ but not totally absent β globin chain production

leads to heterogeneous clinical presentation due to wide variety of mutations

inadequate levels of β globin chains for normal hemoglobin synthesis contributes to the α : β globin chain imbalance

β thalassemia major (aka **Cooley's anemia**)

both β globin genes are severely affected by mutation

most severe form of disease requiring lifelong transfusions

while α globin chains production continues normally

excess of normal α globin chains relative to abnormal or absent β chains

both types of mutation and degree of this imbalance determine clinical phenotype

clinical onset begins at 3 to 6 months when **fetal hemoglobin** production stops and no longer masks abnormality

⇩ Hb A production = **moderate to severe anemia**

some α chains cannot find β chains to pair up with

unpaired α chains form intracellular precipitates which accumulate as **inclusion bodies**

inclusion bodies cause oxidative damage to RBC membrane

⇩ oxygen carrying capacity

hypoxia stimulates erythropoiesis in both bone marrow and extramedullary sites such as liver and spleen

ineffective erythropoiesis

intravascular hemolysis

deformed red blood cells are sequestered in spleen = **splenomegaly**

microcytic hypochromic hemolytic **anemia**

bone marrow expansion causes:
• fractures (especially long bones)
• frontal bossing
• maxillary marrow hyperplasia (chipmunk facies)

stimulates ⇧ iron absorption

hemochromatosis (see map)

abnormal blood smear shows:
• inclusions bodies
• target cells
• bizarre cells
• anisocytosis

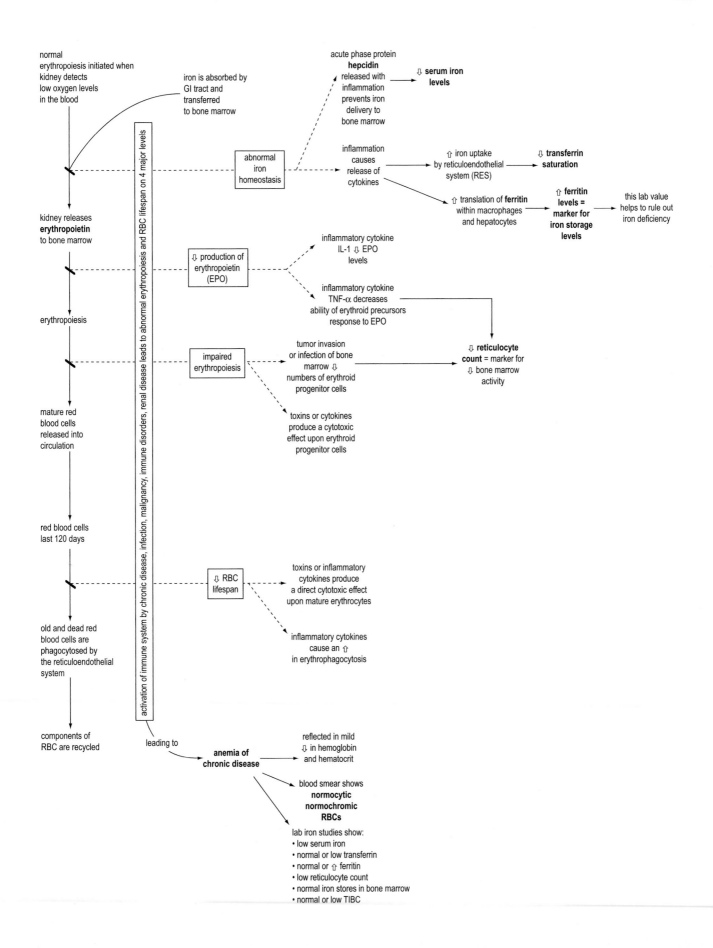

normal
erythropoiesis initiated when
kidney detects
low oxygen levels
in the blood

iron is absorbed by
GI tract and
transferred
to bone marrow

acute phase protein
hepcidin
released with
inflammation
prevents iron
delivery to
bone marrow

⇩ **serum iron
levels**

abnormal
iron
homeostasis

inflammation
causes
release of
cytokines

⇧ iron uptake
by reticuloendothelial
system (RES)

⇩ **transferrin
saturation**

⇧ translation of **ferritin**
within macrophages
and hepatocytes

⇧ **ferritin
levels =
marker for
iron storage
levels**

this lab value
helps to rule out
iron deficiency

kidney releases
erythropoietin
to bone marrow

⇩ production of
erythropoietin
(EPO)

inflammatory cytokine
IL-1 ⇩ EPO
levels

inflammatory cytokine
TNF-α decreases
ability of erythroid precursors
response to EPO

erythropoiesis

impaired
erythropoiesis

tumor invasion
or infection of bone
marrow ⇩
numbers of erythroid
progenitor cells

⇩ **reticulocyte
count** = marker for
⇩ bone marrow
activity

mature red
blood cells
released into
circulation

toxins or cytokines
produce a cytotoxic
effect upon erythroid
progenitor cells

red blood cells
last 120 days

old and dead red
blood cells are
phagocytosed by
the reticuloendothelial
system

⇩ RBC
lifespan

toxins or inflammatory
cytokines produce
a direct cytotoxic effect
upon mature erythrocytes

inflammatory cytokines
cause an ⇧
in erythrophagocytosis

activation of immune system by chronic disease, infection, malignancy, immune disorders, renal disease leads to abnormal erythropoiesis and RBC lifespan on 4 major levels

components of
RBC are recycled

leading to

**anemia of
chronic disease**

reflected in mild
⇩ in hemoglobin
and hematocrit

blood smear shows
**normocytic
normochromic
RBCs**

lab iron studies show:
• low serum iron
• normal or low transferrin
• normal or ⇧ ferritin
• low reticulocyte count
• normal iron stores in bone marrow
• normal or low TIBC

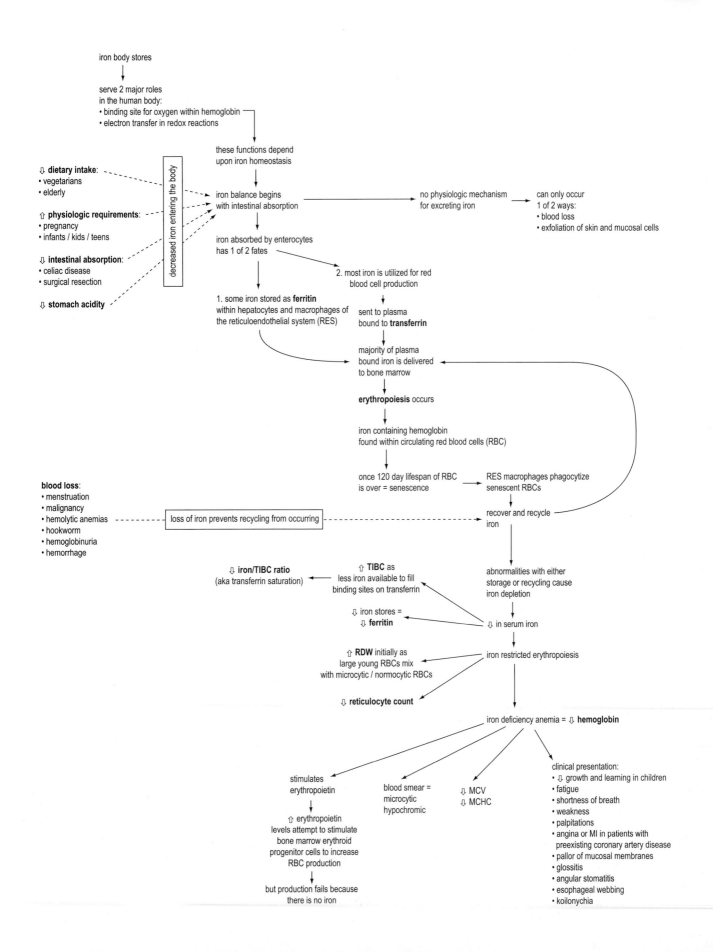

iron body stores

serve 2 major roles
in the human body:
• binding site for oxygen within hemoglobin
• electron transfer in redox reactions

these functions depend
upon iron homeostasis

iron balance begins
with intestinal absorption

no physiologic mechanism
for excreting iron

can only occur
1 of 2 ways:
• blood loss
• exfoliation of skin and mucosal cells

⇩ **dietary intake**:
• vegetarians
• elderly

⇧ **physiologic requirements**:
• pregnancy
• infants / kids / teens

⇩ **intestinal absorption**:
• celiac disease
• surgical resection

⇩ **stomach acidity**

decreased iron entering the body

iron absorbed by enterocytes
has 1 of 2 fates

2. most iron is utilized for red
blood cell production

1. some iron stored as **ferritin**
within hepatocytes and macrophages of
the reticuloendothelial system (RES)

sent to plasma
bound to **transferrin**

majority of plasma
bound iron is delivered
to bone marrow

erythropoiesis occurs

iron containing hemoglobin
found within circulating red blood cells (RBC)

once 120 day lifespan of RBC
is over = senescence

RES macrophages phagocytize
senescent RBCs

blood loss:
• menstruation
• malignancy
• hemolytic anemias
• hookworm
• hemoglobinuria
• hemorrhage

loss of iron prevents recycling from occurring

recover and recycle
iron

⇩ **iron/TIBC ratio**
(aka transferrin saturation)

⇧ TIBC as
less iron available to fill
binding sites on transferrin

abnormalities with either
storage or recycling cause
iron depletion

⇩ iron stores =
⇩ **ferritin**

⇩ in serum iron

⇧ **RDW** initially as
large young RBCs mix
with microcytic / normocytic RBCs

iron restricted erythropoiesis

⇩ **reticulocyte count**

iron deficiency anemia = ⇩ **hemoglobin**

stimulates
erythropoietin

blood smear =
microcytic
hypochromic

⇩ MCV
⇩ MCHC

clinical presentation:
• ⇩ growth and learning in children
• fatigue
• shortness of breath
• weakness
• palpitations
• angina or MI in patients with
  preexisting coronary artery disease
• pallor of mucosal membranes
• glossitis
• angular stomatitis
• esophageal webbing
• koilonychia

⇧ erythropoietin
levels attempt to stimulate
bone marrow erythroid
progenitor cells to increase
RBC production

but production fails because
there is no iron

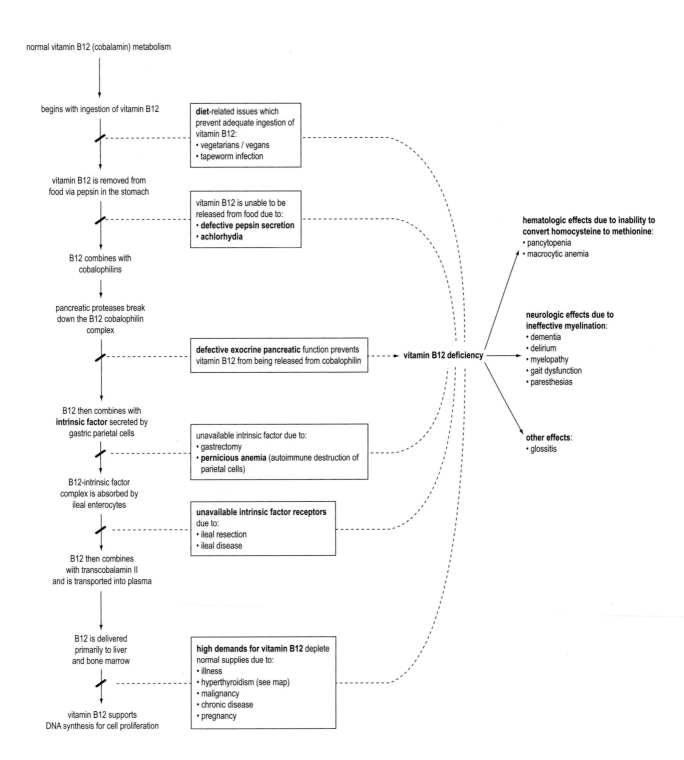

normal vitamin B12 (cobalamin) metabolism

begins with ingestion of vitamin B12

diet-related issues which
prevent adequate ingestion of
vitamin B12:
• vegetarians / vegans
• tapeworm infection

vitamin B12 is removed from
food via pepsin in the stomach

vitamin B12 is unable to be
released from food due to:
• **defective pepsin secretion**
• **achlorhydia**

B12 combines with
cobalophilins

pancreatic proteases break
down the B12 cobalophilin
complex

defective exocrine pancreatic function prevents
vitamin B12 from being released from cobalophilin

B12 then combines with
intrinsic factor secreted by
gastric parietal cells

unavailable intrinsic factor due to:
• gastrectomy
• **pernicious anemia** (autoimmune destruction of
  parietal cells)

B12-intrinsic factor
complex is absorbed by
ileal enterocytes

unavailable intrinsic factor receptors
due to:
• ileal resection
• ileal disease

B12 then combines
with transcobalamin II
and is transported into plasma

B12 is delivered
primarily to liver
and bone marrow

high demands for vitamin B12 deplete
normal supplies due to:
• illness
• hyperthyroidism (see map)
• malignancy
• chronic disease
• pregnancy

vitamin B12 supports
DNA synthesis for cell proliferation

vitamin B12 deficiency

**hematologic effects due to inability to
convert homocysteine to methionine:**
• pancytopenia
• macrocytic anemia

**neurologic effects due to
ineffective myelination:**
• dementia
• delirium
• myelopathy
• gait dysfunction
• paresthesias

other effects:
• glossitis

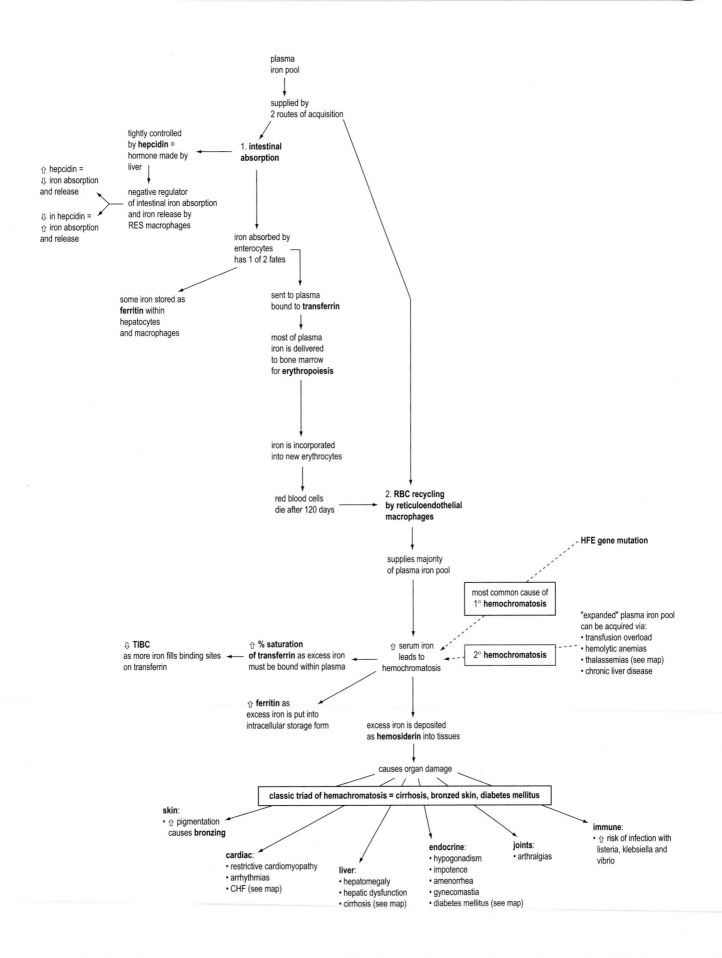

plasma
iron pool

supplied by
2 routes of acquisition

tightly controlled
by **hepcidin** =
hormone made by
liver

**1. intestinal
absorption**

⇑ hepcidin =
⇓ iron absorption
and release

negative regulator
of intestinal iron absorption
and iron release by
RES macrophages

⇓ in hepcidin =
⇑ iron absorption
and release

iron absorbed by
enterocytes
has 1 of 2 fates

some iron stored as
ferritin within
hepatocytes
and macrophages

sent to plasma
bound to **transferrin**

most of plasma
iron is delivered
to bone marrow
for **erythropoiesis**

iron is incorporated
into new erythrocytes

red blood cells
die after 120 days

**2. RBC recycling
by reticuloendothelial
macrophages**

supplies majority
of plasma iron pool

HFE gene mutation

most common cause of
1° **hemochromatosis**

"expanded" plasma iron pool
can be acquired via:
• transfusion overload
• hemolytic anemias
• thalassemias (see map)
• chronic liver disease

⇓ TIBC
as more iron fills binding sites
on transferrin

⇑ **% saturation
of transferrin** as excess iron
must be bound within plasma

⇑ serum iron
leads to
hemochromatosis

2° **hemochromatosis**

⇑ **ferritin** as
excess iron is put into
intracellular storage form

excess iron is deposited
as **hemosiderin** into tissues

causes organ damage

classic triad of hemachromatosis = cirrhosis, bronzed skin, diabetes mellitus

skin:
• ⇑ pigmentation
causes **bronzing**

cardiac:
• restrictive cardiomyopathy
• arrhythmias
• CHF (see map)

liver:
• hepatomegaly
• hepatic dysfunction
• cirrhosis (see map)

endocrine:
• hypogonadism
• impotence
• amenorrhea
• gynecomastia
• diabetes mellitus (see map)

joints:
• arthralgias

immune:
• ⇑ risk of infection with
listeria, klebsiella and
vibrio

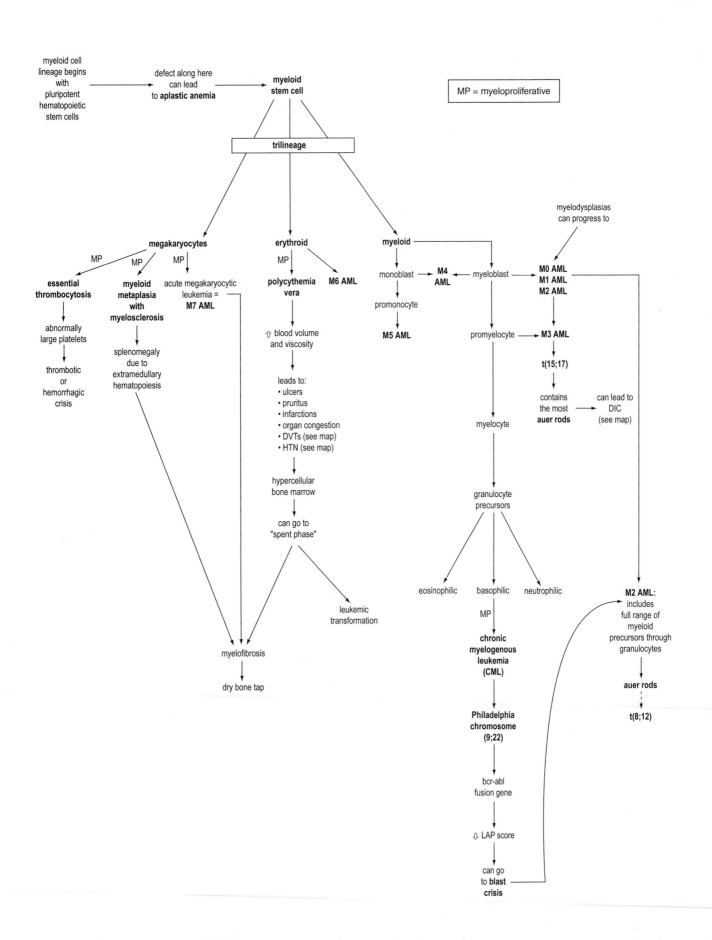

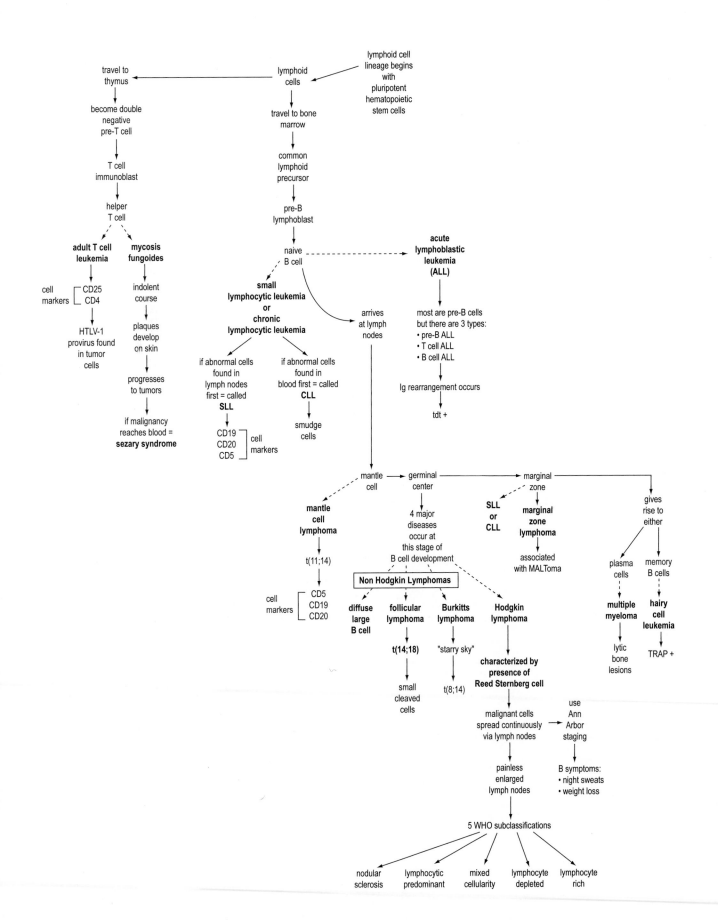

Gastrointestinal Disorders

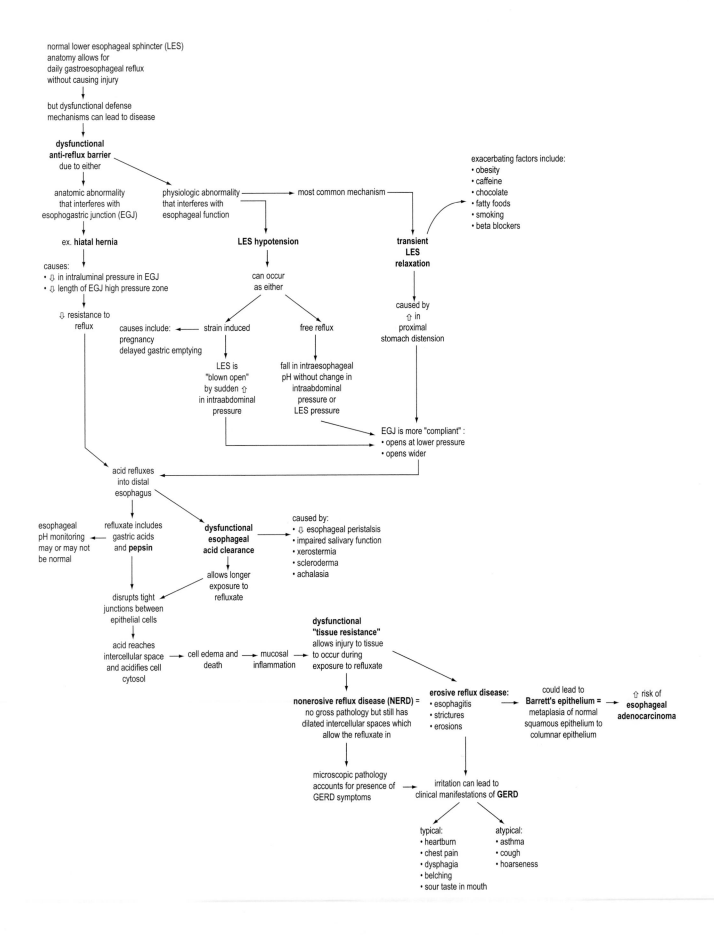

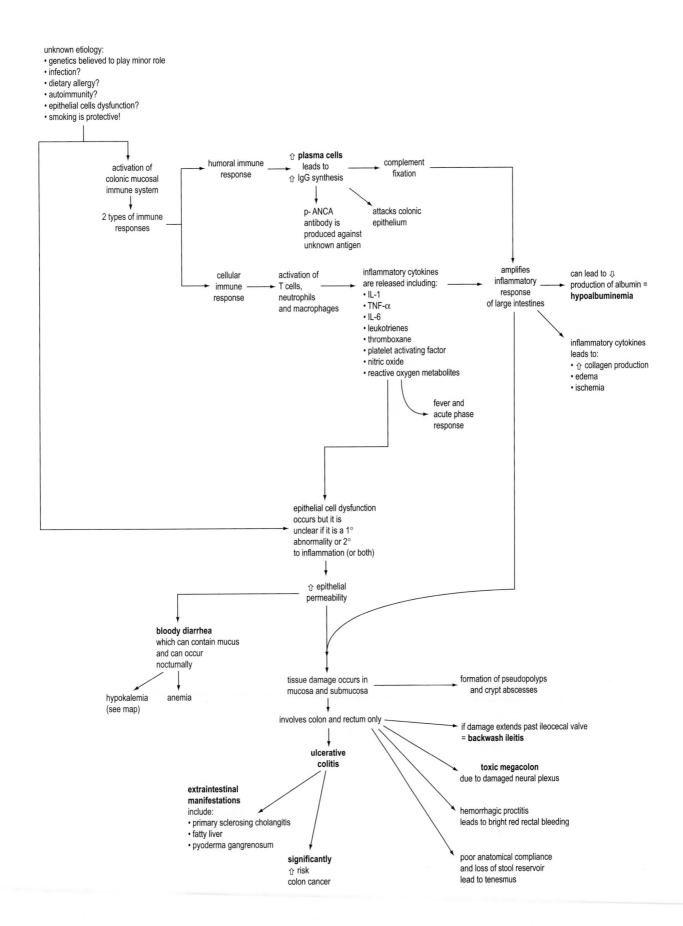

unknown etiology:
• genetics believed to play minor role
• infection?
• dietary allergy?
• autoimmunity?
• epithelial cells dysfunction?
• smoking is protective!

activation of
colonic mucosal
immune system

2 types of immune
responses

humoral immune
response

⇧ **plasma cells**
leads to
⇧ IgG synthesis

complement
fixation

p- ANCA
antibody is
produced against
unknown antigen

attacks colonic
epithelium

cellular
immune
response

activation of
T cells,
neutrophils
and macrophages

inflammatory cytokines
are released including:
• IL-1
• TNF-α
• IL-6
• leukotrienes
• thromboxane
• platelet activating factor
• nitric oxide
• reactive oxygen metabolites

amplifies
inflammatory
response
of large intestines

can lead to ⇩
production of albumin =
hypoalbuminemia

inflammatory cytokines
leads to:
• ⇧ collagen production
• edema
• ischemia

fever and
acute phase
response

epithelial cell dysfunction
occurs but it is
unclear if it is a 1°
abnormality or 2°
to inflammation (or both)

⇧ epithelial
permeability

bloody diarrhea
which can contain mucus
and can occur
nocturnally

hypokalemia
(see map)

anemia

tissue damage occurs in
mucosa and submucosa

formation of pseudopolyps
and crypt abscesses

involves colon and rectum only

if damage extends past ileocecal valve
= **backwash ileitis**

**ulcerative
colitis**

toxic megacolon
due to damaged neural plexus

**extraintestinal
manifestations**
include:
• primary sclerosing cholangitis
• fatty liver
• pyoderma gangrenosum

hemorrhagic proctitis
leads to bright red rectal bleeding

significantly
⇧ risk
colon cancer

poor anatomical compliance
and loss of stool reservoir
lead to tenesmus

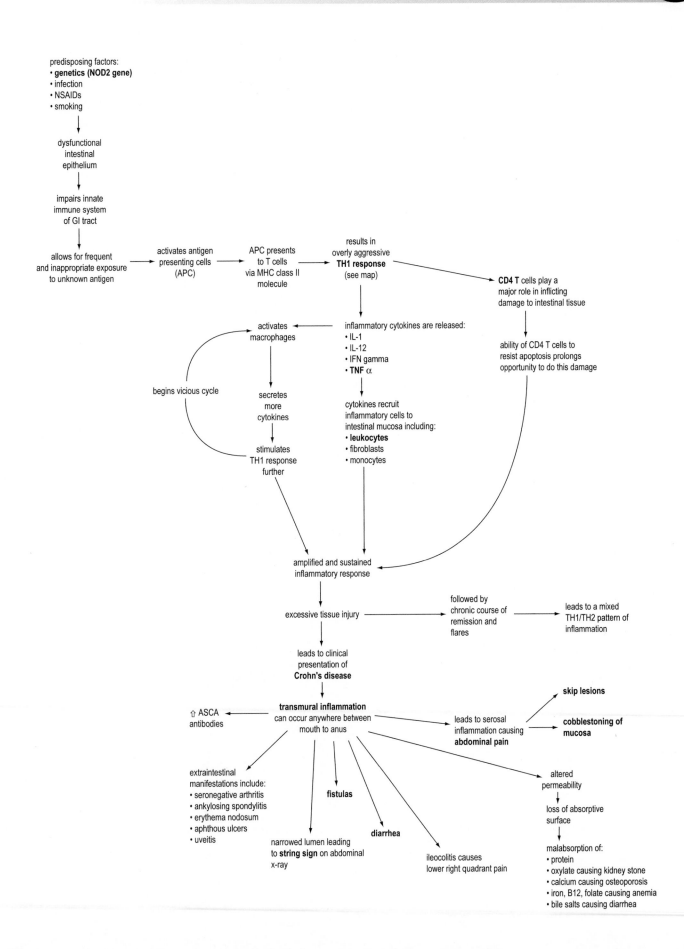

predisposing factors:
• **genetics (NOD2 gene)**
• infection
• NSAIDs
• smoking

dysfunctional intestinal epithelium

impairs innate immune system of GI tract

allows for frequent and inappropriate exposure to unknown antigen → activates antigen presenting cells (APC) → APC presents to T cells via MHC class II molecule → results in overly aggressive **TH1 response** (see map)

CD4 T cells play a major role in inflicting damage to intestinal tissue

ability of CD4 T cells to resist apoptosis prolongs opportunity to do this damage

inflammatory cytokines are released:
• IL-1
• IL-12
• IFN gamma
• **TNF** α

activates macrophages

begins vicious cycle

secretes more cytokines

stimulates TH1 response further

cytokines recruit inflammatory cells to intestinal mucosa including:
• **leukocytes**
• fibroblasts
• monocytes

amplified and sustained inflammatory response

excessive tissue injury → followed by chronic course of remission and flares → leads to a mixed TH1/TH2 pattern of inflammation

leads to clinical presentation of **Crohn's disease**

transmural inflammation can occur anywhere between mouth to anus

⇧ ASCA antibodies

leads to serosal inflammation causing **abdominal pain**

skip lesions

cobblestoning of mucosa

extraintestinal manifestations include:
• seronegative arthritis
• ankylosing spondylitis
• erythema nodosum
• aphthous ulcers
• uveitis

fistulas

diarrhea

altered permeability

loss of absorptive surface

narrowed lumen leading to **string sign** on abdominal x-ray

ileocolitis causes lower right quadrant pain

malabsorption of:
• protein
• oxalate causing kidney stone
• calcium causing osteoporosis
• iron, B12, folate causing anemia
• bile salts causing diarrhea

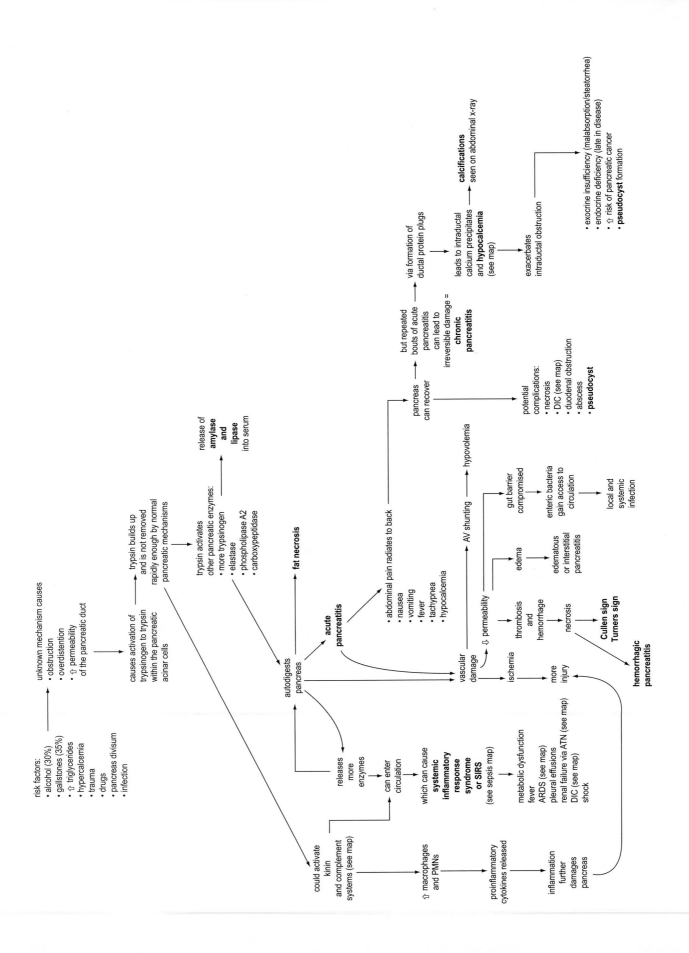

risk factors:
• alcohol (30%)
• gallstones (35%)
• ⇧ triglycerides
• hypercalcemia
• trauma
• drugs
• pancreas divisum
• infection

unknown mechanism causes
• obstruction
• overdistention
• ⇧ permeability
of the pancreatic duct

causes activation of trypsinogen to trypsin within the pancreatic acinar cells

trypsin builds up and is not removed rapidly enough by normal pancreatic mechanisms

release of amylase and lipase into serum

trypsin activates other pancreatic enzymes:
• more trypsinogen
• elastase
• phospholipase A2
• carboxypeptidase

fat necrosis

autodigests pancreas

acute pancreatitis

• abdominal pain radiates to back
• nausea
• vomiting
• fever
• tachypnea
• hypocalcemia

releases more enzymes

can enter circulation

which can cause systemic inflammatory response syndrome or SIRS (see sepsis map)

metabolic dysfunction
fever
ARDS (see map)
pleural effusions
renal failure via ATN (see map)
DIC (see map)
shock

could activate kinin and complement systems (see map)

⇧ macrophages and PMNs

proinflammatory cytokines released

inflammation further damages pancreas

vascular damage

ischemia

more injury

⇧ permeability

thrombosis and hemorrhage

necrosis

Cullen sign
Turners sign

hemorrhagic pancreatitis

AV shunting → hypovolemia

edema → edematous or interstitial pancreatitis

gut barrier compromised → enteric bacteria gain access to circulation → local and systemic infection

pancreas can recover

but repeated bouts of acute pancreatitis can lead to irreversible damage = chronic pancreatitis

via formation of ductal protein plugs

leads to intraductal calcium precipitates and hypocalcemia (see map)

calcifications seen on abdominal x-ray

exacerbates intraductal obstruction

• exocrine insufficiency (malabsorption/steatorrhea)
• endocrine deficiency (late in disease)
• ⇧ risk of pancreatic cancer
• pseudocyst formation

potential complications:
• necrosis
• DIC (see map)
• duodenal obstruction
• abscess
• pseudocyst

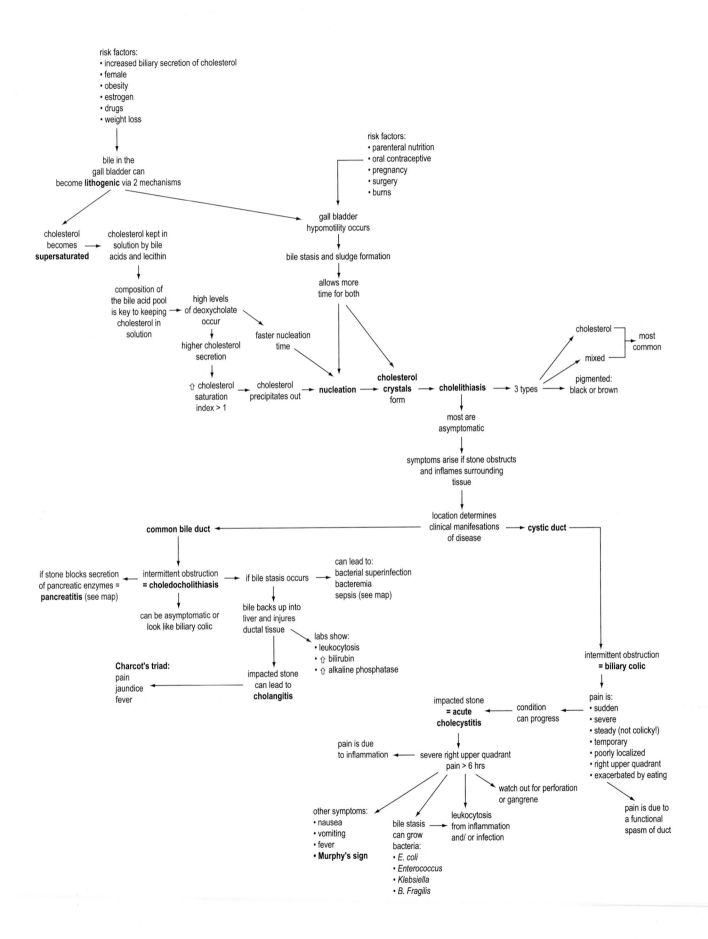

Liver Disorders

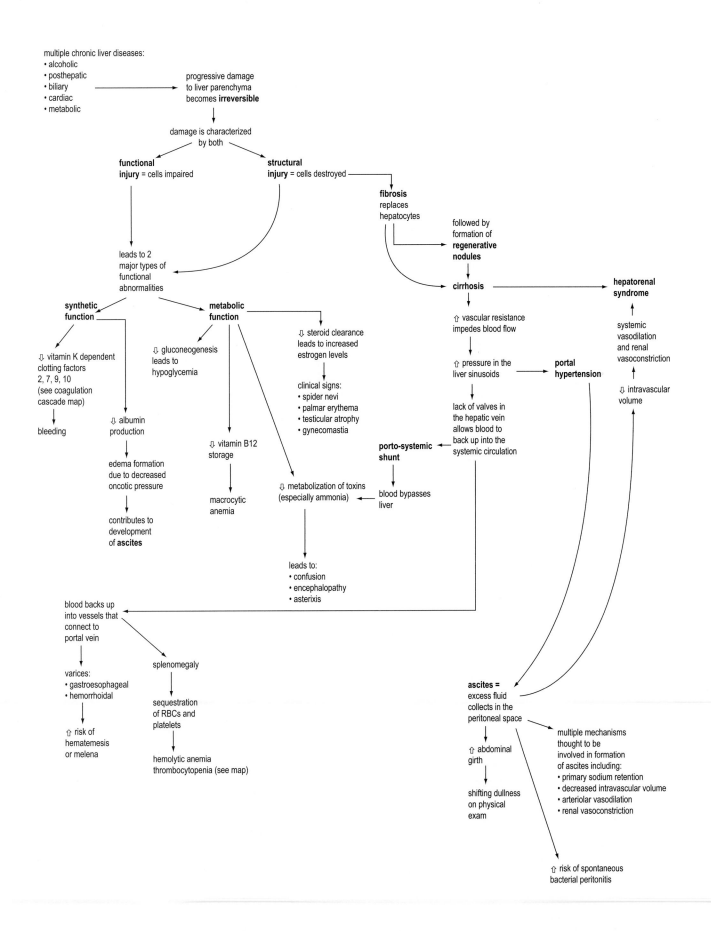

multiple chronic liver diseases:
• alcoholic
• posthepatic
• biliary
• cardiac
• metabolic

progressive damage to liver parenchyma becomes **irreversible**

damage is characterized by both

functional injury = cells impaired

structural injury = cells destroyed

fibrosis replaces hepatocytes

followed by formation of **regenerative nodules**

cirrhosis

hepatorenal syndrome

leads to 2 major types of functional abnormalities

synthetic function

metabolic function

⇩ vascular resistance impedes blood flow

systemic vasodilation and renal vasoconstriction

⇩ vitamin K dependent clotting factors 2, 7, 9, 10 (see coagulation cascade map)

⇩ gluconeogenesis leads to hypoglycemia

⇩ steroid clearance leads to increased estrogen levels

⇧ pressure in the liver sinusoids

portal hypertension

⇩ intravascular volume

bleeding

clinical signs:
• spider nevi
• palmar erythema
• testicular atrophy
• gynecomastia

lack of valves in the hepatic vein allows blood to back up into the systemic circulation

⇩ albumin production

⇩ vitamin B12 storage

porto-systemic shunt

edema formation due to decreased oncotic pressure

macrocytic anemia

⇩ metabolization of toxins (especially ammonia)

blood bypasses liver

contributes to development **of ascites**

leads to:
• confusion
• encephalopathy
• asterixis

blood backs up into vessels that connect to portal vein

varices:
• gastroesophageal
• hemorrhoidal

splenomegaly

⇧ risk of hematemesis or melena

sequestration of RBCs and platelets

hemolytic anemia thrombocytopenia (see map)

ascites = excess fluid collects in the peritoneal space

multiple mechanisms thought to be involved in formation of ascites including:
• primary sodium retention
• decreased intravascular volume
• arteriolar vasodilation
• renal vasoconstriction

⇧ abdominal girth

shifting dullness on physical exam

⇧ risk of spontaneous bacterial peritonitis

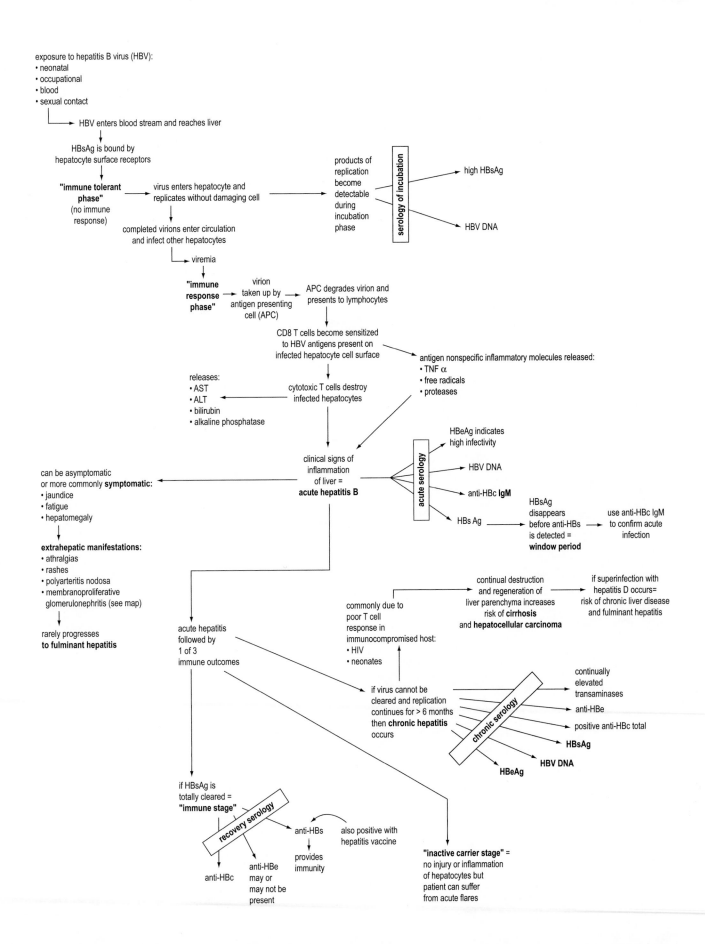

exposure to hepatitis B virus (HBV):
• neonatal
• occupational
• blood
• sexual contact

HBV enters blood stream and reaches liver

HBsAg is bound by
hepatocyte surface receptors

**"immune tolerant
phase"**
(no immune
response)

virus enters hepatocyte and
replicates without damaging cell

completed virions enter circulation
and infect other hepatocytes

viremia

products of
replication
become
detectable
during
incubation
phase

serology of incubation

high HBsAg

HBV DNA

**"immune
response
phase"**

virion
taken up by
antigen presenting
cell (APC)

APC degrades virion and
presents to lymphocytes

CD8 T cells become sensitized
to HBV antigens present on
infected hepatocyte cell surface

antigen nonspecific inflammatory molecules released:
• TNF α
• free radicals
• proteases

releases:
• AST
• ALT
• bilirubin
• alkaline phosphatase

cytotoxic T cells destroy
infected hepatocytes

clinical signs of
inflammation
of liver =
acute hepatitis B

acute serology

HBeAg indicates
high infectivity

HBV DNA

anti-HBc **IgM**

HBs Ag

HBsAg
disappears
before anti-HBs
is detected =
window period

use anti-HBc IgM
to confirm acute
infection

can be asymptomatic
or more commonly **symptomatic:**
• jaundice
• fatigue
• hepatomegaly

extrahepatic manifestations:
• athralgias
• rashes
• polyarteritis nodosa
• membranoproliferative
  glomerulonephritis (see map)

rarely progresses
to fulminant hepatitis

acute hepatitis
followed by
1 of 3
immune outcomes

commonly due to
poor T cell
response in
immunocompromised host:
• HIV
• neonates

continual destruction
and regeneration of
liver parenchyma increases
risk of **cirrhosis**
and **hepatocellular carcinoma**

if superinfection with
hepatitis D occurs=
risk of chronic liver disease
and fulminant hepatitis

if virus cannot be
cleared and replication
continues for > 6 months
then **chronic hepatitis**
occurs

chronic serology

continually
elevated
transaminases

anti-HBe

positive anti-HBc total

HBsAg

HBV DNA

HBeAg

if HBsAg is
totally cleared =
"immune stage"

recovery serology

anti-HBs

also positive with
hepatitis vaccine

provides
immunity

anti-HBc

anti-HBe
may or
may not be
present

"inactive carrier stage" =
no injury or inflammation
of hepatocytes but
patient can suffer
from acute flares

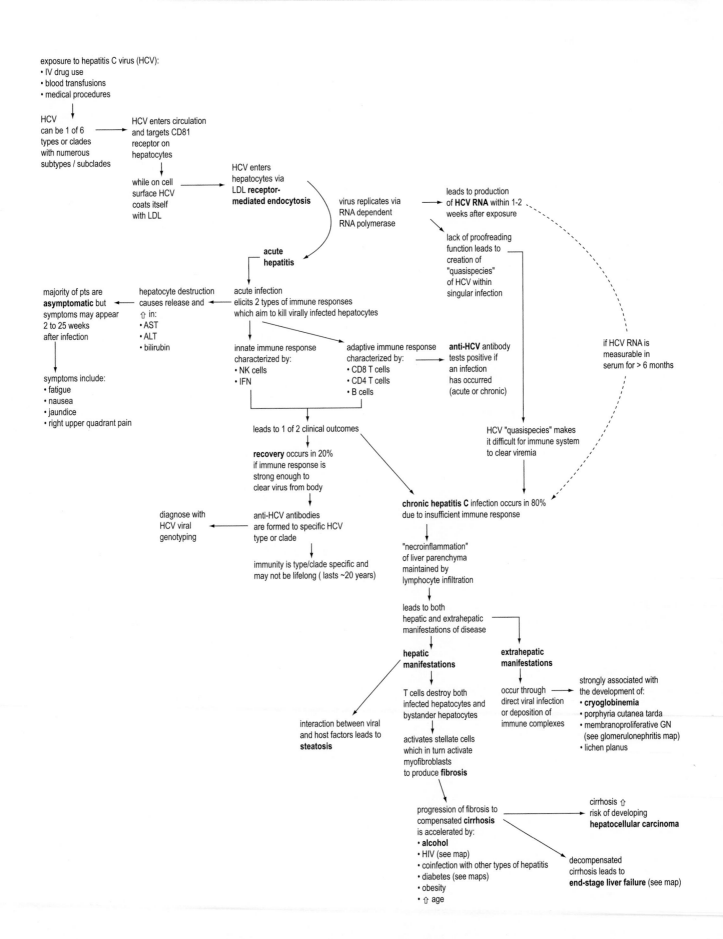

exposure to hepatitis C virus (HCV):
• IV drug use
• blood transfusions
• medical procedures

HCV
can be 1 of 6
types or clades
with numerous
subtypes / subclades

HCV enters circulation
and targets CD81
receptor on
hepatocytes

while on cell
surface HCV
coats itself
with LDL

HCV enters
hepatocytes via
LDL **receptor-
mediated endocytosis**

virus replicates via
RNA dependent
RNA polymerase

leads to production
of **HCV RNA** within 1-2
weeks after exposure

lack of proofreading
function leads to
creation of
"quasispecies"
of HCV within
singular infection

**acute
hepatitis**

majority of pts are
asymptomatic but
symptoms may appear
2 to 25 weeks
after infection

hepatocyte destruction
causes release and
⇧ in:
• AST
• ALT
• bilirubin

acute infection
elicits 2 types of immune responses
which aim to kill virally infected hepatocytes

if HCV RNA is
measurable in
serum for > 6 months

symptoms include:
• fatigue
• nausea
• jaundice
• right upper quadrant pain

innate immune response
characterized by:
• NK cells
• IFN

adaptive immune response
characterized by:
• CD8 T cells
• CD4 T cells
• B cells

anti-HCV antibody
tests positive if
an infection
has occurred
(acute or chronic)

leads to 1 of 2 clinical outcomes

HCV "quasispecies" makes
it difficult for immune system
to clear viremia

recovery occurs in 20%
if immune response is
strong enough to
clear virus from body

diagnose with
HCV viral
genotyping

anti-HCV antibodies
are formed to specific HCV
type or clade

chronic hepatitis C infection occurs in 80%
due to insufficient immune response

immunity is type/clade specific and
may not be lifelong (lasts ~20 years)

"necroinflammation"
of liver parenchyma
maintained by
lymphocyte infiltration

leads to both
hepatic and extrahepatic
manifestations of disease

**hepatic
manifestations**

**extrahepatic
manifestations**

T cells destroy both
infected hepatocytes and
bystander hepatocytes

occur through
direct viral infection
or deposition of
immune complexes

strongly associated with
the development of:
• **cryoglobinemia**
• porphyria cutanea tarda
• membranoproliferative GN
  (see glomerulonephritis map)
• lichen planus

interaction between viral
and host factors leads to
steatosis

activates stellate cells
which in turn activate
myofibroblasts
to produce **fibrosis**

progression of fibrosis to
compensated **cirrhosis**
is accelerated by:
• **alcohol**
• HIV (see map)
• coinfection with other types of hepatitis
• diabetes (see maps)
• obesity
• ⇧ age

cirrhosis ⇧
risk of developing
hepatocellular carcinoma

decompensated
cirrhosis leads to
end-stage liver failure (see map)

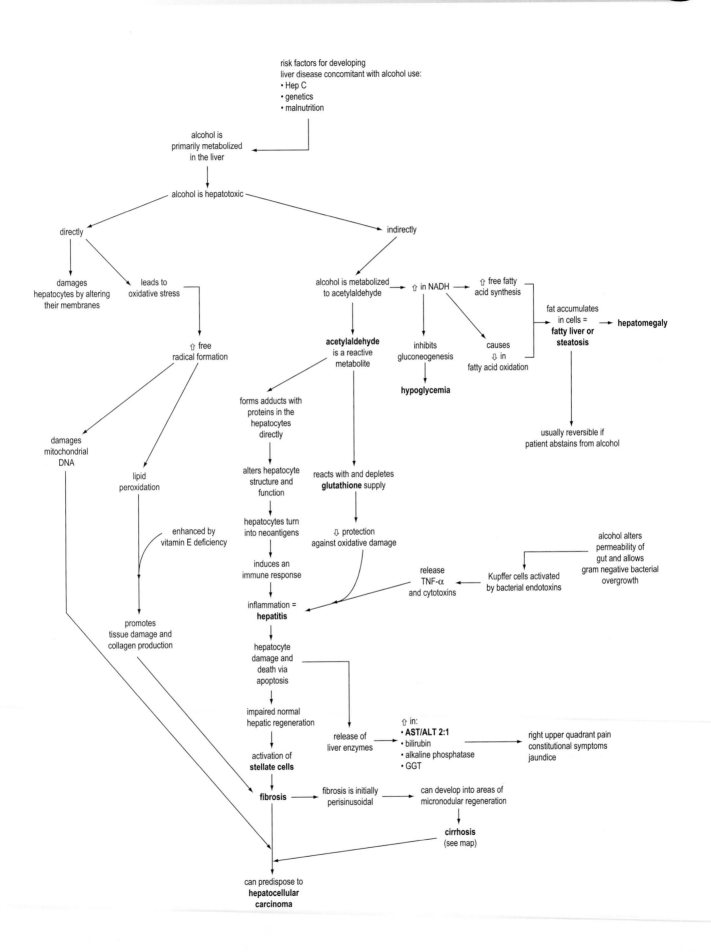

Renal Disorders

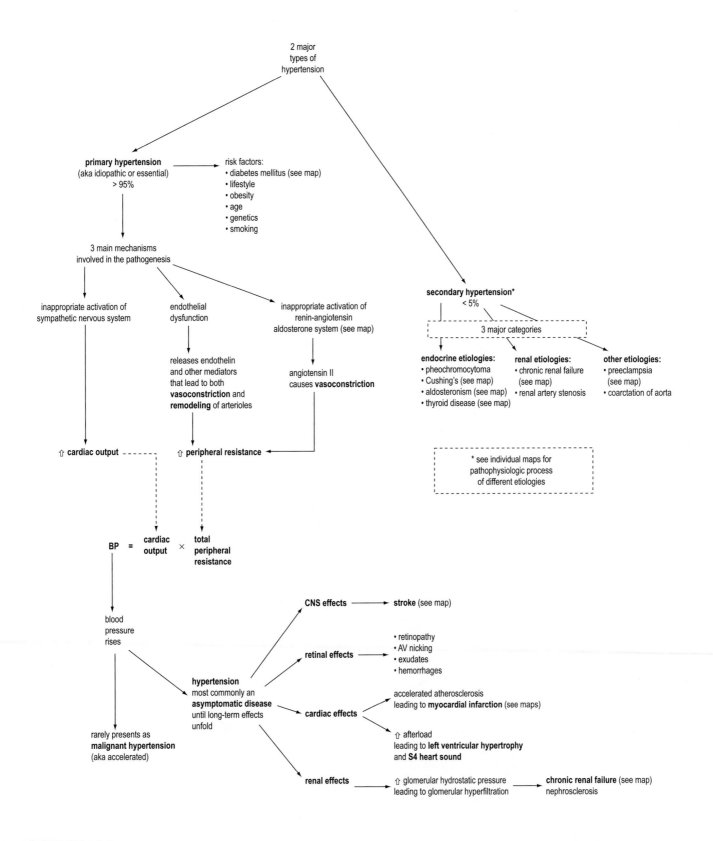

2 major
types of
hypertension

primary hypertension
(aka idiopathic or essential)
> 95%

risk factors:
• diabetes mellitus (see map)
• lifestyle
• obesity
• age
• genetics
• smoking

3 main mechanisms
involved in the pathogenesis

inappropriate activation of
sympathetic nervous system

endothelial
dysfunction

inappropriate activation of
renin-angiotensin
aldosterone system (see map)

secondary hypertension*
< 5%

3 major categories

endocrine etiologies:
• pheochromocytoma
• Cushing's (see map)
• aldosteronism (see map)
• thyroid disease (see map)

renal etiologies:
• chronic renal failure
  (see map)
• renal artery stenosis

other etiologies:
• preeclampsia
  (see map)
• coarctation of aorta

releases endothelin
and other mediators
that lead to both
vasoconstriction and
remodeling of arterioles

angiotensin II
causes **vasoconstriction**

⇧ **cardiac output**

⇧ **peripheral resistance**

* see individual maps for
pathophysiologic process
of different etiologies

BP = cardiac
output × total
peripheral
resistance

blood
pressure
rises

rarely presents as
malignant hypertension
(aka accelerated)

hypertension
most commonly an
asymptomatic disease
until long-term effects
unfold

CNS effects ⟶ **stroke** (see map)

retinal effects
• retinopathy
• AV nicking
• exudates
• hemorrhages

cardiac effects
accelerated atherosclerosis
leading to **myocardial infarction** (see maps)

⇧ afterload
leading to **left ventricular hypertrophy**
and **S4 heart sound**

renal effects
⇧ glomerular hydrostatic pressure
leading to glomerular hyperfiltration ⟶ **chronic renal failure** (see map)
nephrosclerosis

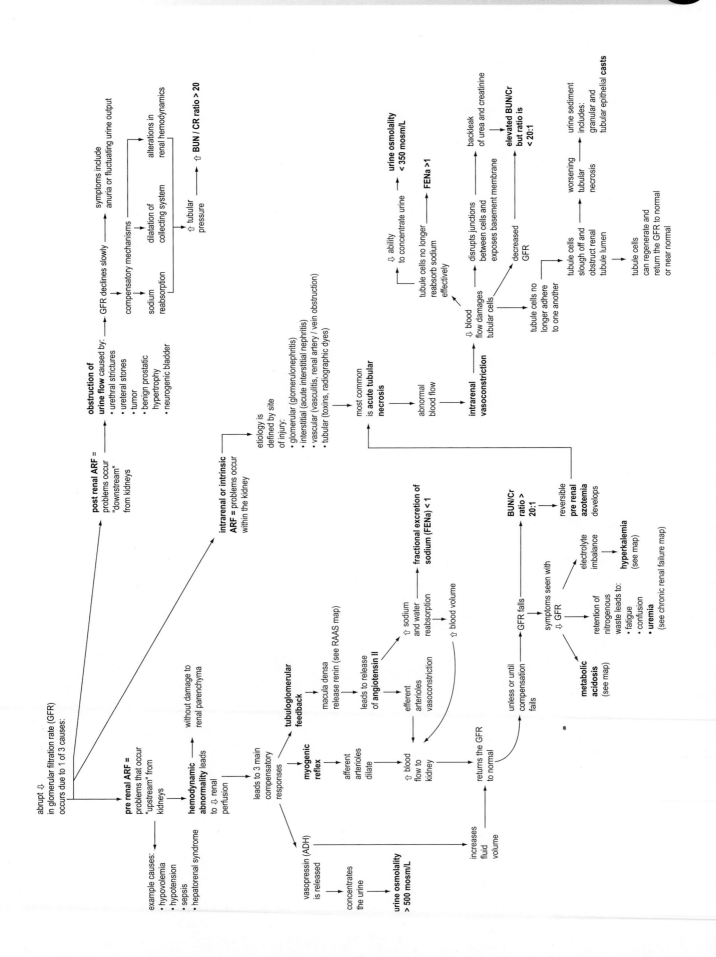

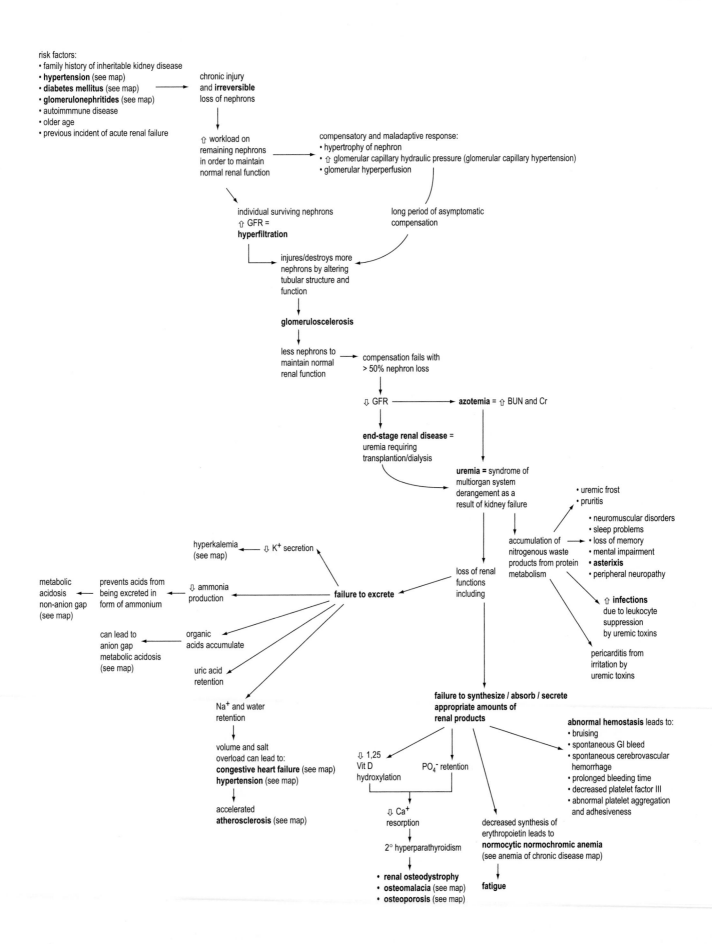

risk factors:
• family history of inheritable kidney disease
• **hypertension** (see map)
• **diabetes mellitus** (see map)
• **glomerulonephritides** (see map)
• autoimmmune disease
• older age
• previous incident of acute renal failure

chronic injury and **irreversible** loss of nephrons

⇧ workload on remaining nephrons in order to maintain normal renal function

compensatory and maladaptive response:
• hypertrophy of nephron
• ⇧ glomerular capillary hydraulic pressure (glomerular capillary hypertension)
• glomerular hyperperfusion

individual surviving nephrons ⇧ GFR = **hyperfiltration**

long period of asymptomatic compensation

injures/destroys more nephrons by altering tubular structure and function

glomerulosclerosis

less nephrons to maintain normal renal function

compensation fails with > 50% nephron loss

⇩ GFR ⟶ **azotemia** = ⇧ BUN and Cr

end-stage renal disease = uremia requiring transplantion/dialysis

uremia = syndrome of multiorgan system derangement as a result of kidney failure

accumulation of nitrogenous waste products from protein metabolism

• uremic frost
• pruritis

• neuromuscular disorders
• sleep problems
• loss of memory
• mental impairment
• **asterixis**
• peripheral neuropathy

⇧ **infections** due to leukocyte suppression by uremic toxins

pericarditis from irritation by uremic toxins

loss of renal functions including

failure to excrete

hyperkalemia (see map) ⟵ ⇩ K⁺ secretion

metabolic acidosis non-anion gap (see map) ⟵ prevents acids from being excreted in form of ammonium ⟵ ⇩ ammonia production

can lead to anion gap metabolic acidosis (see map) ⟵ organic acids accumulate

uric acid retention

Na⁺ and water retention

volume and salt overload can lead to:
congestive heart failure (see map)
hypertension (see map)

accelerated **atherosclerosis** (see map)

failure to synthesize / absorb / secrete appropriate amounts of renal products

⇩ 1,25 Vit D hydroxylation

PO₄⁻ retention

⇩ Ca⁺ resorption

2° hyperparathyroidism

• **renal osteodystrophy**
• **osteomalacia** (see map)
• **osteoporosis** (see map)

abnormal hemostasis leads to:
• bruising
• spontaneous GI bleed
• spontaneous cerebrovascular hemorrhage
• prolonged bleeding time
• decreased platelet factor III
• abnormal platelet aggregation and adhesiveness

decreased synthesis of erythropoietin leads to **normocytic normochromic anemia** (see anemia of chronic disease map)

fatigue

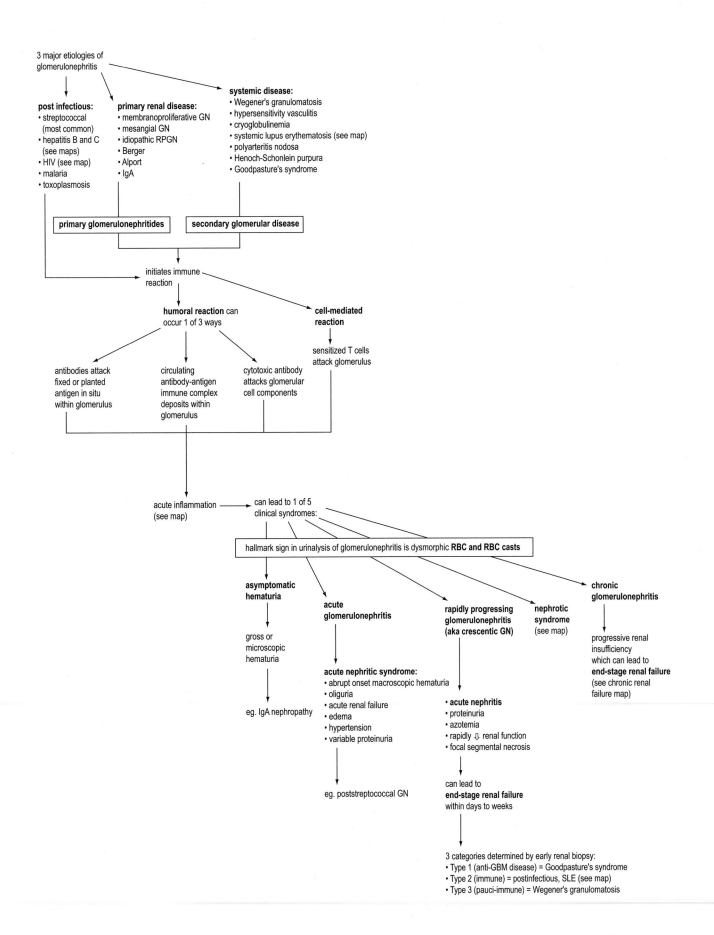

3 major etiologies of glomerulonephritis

post infectious:
• streptococcal (most common)
• hepatitis B and C (see maps)
• HIV (see map)
• malaria
• toxoplasmosis

primary renal disease:
• membranoproliferative GN
• mesangial GN
• idiopathic RPGN
• Berger
• Alport
• IgA

systemic disease:
• Wegener's granulomatosis
• hypersensitivity vasculitis
• cryoglobulinemia
• systemic lupus erythematosis (see map)
• polyarteritis nodosa
• Henoch-Schonlein purpura
• Goodpasture's syndrome

primary glomerulonephritides

secondary glomerular disease

initiates immune reaction

humoral reaction can occur 1 of 3 ways

cell-mediated reaction

sensitized T cells attack glomerulus

antibodies attack fixed or planted antigen in situ within glomerulus

circulating antibody-antigen immune complex deposits within glomerulus

cytotoxic antibody attacks glomerular cell components

acute inflammation (see map)

can lead to 1 of 5 clinical syndromes:

hallmark sign in urinalysis of glomerulonephritis is dysmorphic **RBC and RBC casts**

asymptomatic hematuria

gross or microscopic hematuria

eg. IgA nephropathy

acute glomerulonephritis

acute nephritic syndrome:
• abrupt onset macroscopic hematuria
• oliguria
• acute renal failure
• edema
• hypertension
• variable proteinuria

eg. poststreptococcal GN

rapidly progressing glomerulonephritis (aka crescentic GN)

• **acute nephritis**
• proteinuria
• azotemia
• rapidly ⇩ renal function
• focal segmental necrosis

can lead to
end-stage renal failure
within days to weeks

3 categories determined by early renal biopsy:
• Type 1 (anti-GBM disease) = Goodpasture's syndrome
• Type 2 (immune) = postinfectious, SLE (see map)
• Type 3 (pauci-immune) = Wegener's granulomatosis

nephrotic syndrome (see map)

chronic glomerulonephritis

progressive renal insufficiency which can lead to
end-stage renal failure (see chronic renal failure map)

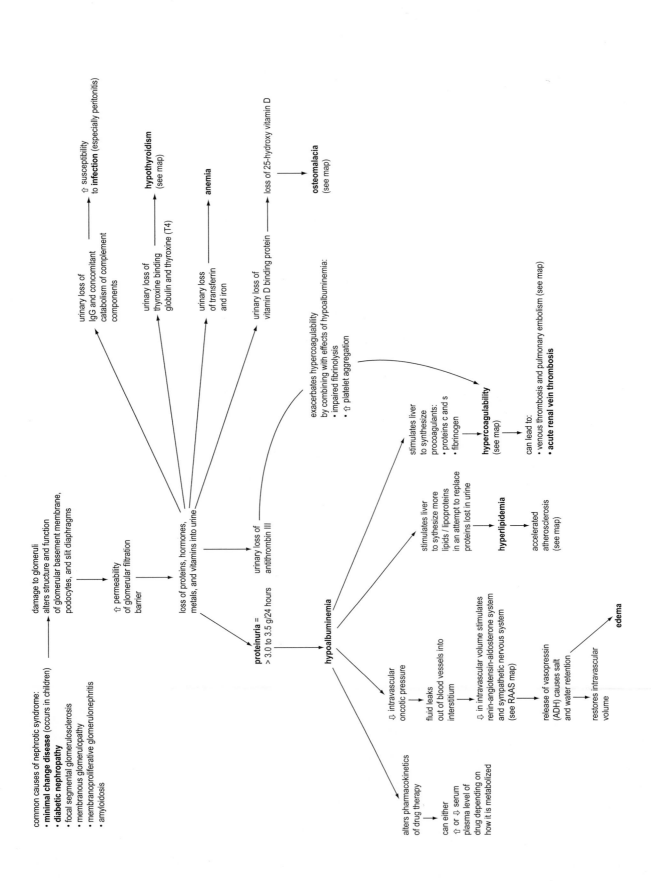

common causes of nephrotic syndrome:
• **minimal change disease** (occurs in children)
• **diabetic nephropathy**
• focal segmental glomerulosclerosis
• membranous glomerulopathy
• membranoproliferative glomerulonephritis
• amyloidosis

damage to glomeruli
alters structure and function
of glomerular basement membrane,
podocytes, and slit diaphragms

⇧ permeability
of glomerular filtration
barrier

loss of proteins, hormones,
metals, and vitamins into urine

urinary loss of
IgG and concomitant
catabolism of complement
components

⇧ susceptibility
to **infection** (especially peritonitis)

urinary loss of
thyroxine binding
globulin and thyroxine (T4)

hypothyroidism
(see map)

urinary loss
of transferrin
and iron

anemia

urinary loss of
vitamin D binding protein

loss of 25-hydroxy vitamin D

osteomalacia
(see map)

urinary loss of
antithrombin III

proteinuria =
> 3.0 to 3.5 g/24 hours

hypoalbuminemia

exacerbates hypercoagulability
by combining with effects of hypoalbuminemia:
• impaired fibrinolysis
• ⇧ platelet aggregation

stimulates liver
to synthesize
procoagulants:
• proteins c and s
• fibrinogen

hypercoagulability
(see map)

can lead to:
• venous thrombosis and pulmonary embolism (see map)
• **acute renal vein thrombosis**

stimulates liver
to sythesize more
lipids / lipoproteins
in an attempt to replace
proteins lost in urine

hyperlipidemia

accelerated
atherosclerosis
(see map)

⇩ intravascular
oncotic pressure

fluid leaks
out of blood vessels into
interstitium

⇩ in intravascular volume stimulates
renin-angiotensin-aldosterone system
and sympathetic nervous system
(see RAAS map)

release of vasopressin
(ADH) causes salt
and water retention

restores intravascular
volume

edema

alters pharmacokinetics
of drug therapy

can either
⇧ or ⇩ serum
plasma level of
drug depending on
how it is metabolized

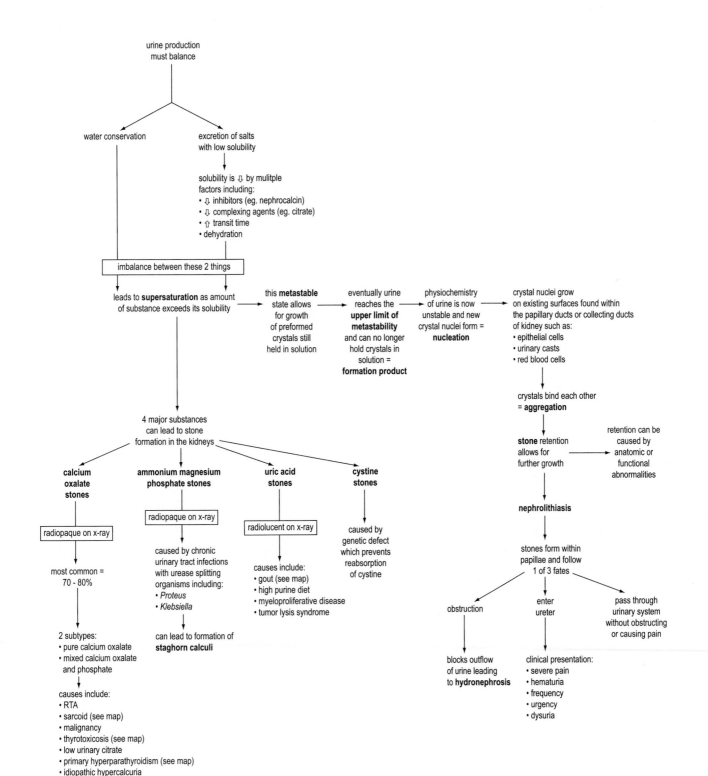

urine production
must balance

water conservation

excretion of salts
with low solubility

solubility is ⇩ by mulitple
factors including:
• ⇩ inhibitors (eg. nephrocalcin)
• ⇩ complexing agents (eg. citrate)
• ⇧ transit time
• dehydration

imbalance between these 2 things

leads to **supersaturation** as amount
of substance exceeds its solubility

this **metastable**
state allows
for growth
of preformed
crystals still
held in solution

eventually urine
reaches the
**upper limit of
metastability**
and can no longer
hold crystals in
solution =
formation product

physiochemistry
of urine is now
unstable and new
crystal nuclei form =
nucleation

crystal nuclei grow
on existing surfaces found within
the papillary ducts or collecting ducts
of kidney such as:
• epithelial cells
• urinary casts
• red blood cells

crystals bind each other
= **aggregation**

stone retention
allows for
further growth

retention can be
caused by
anatomic or
functional
abnormalities

nephrolithiasis

stones form within
papillae and follow
1 of 3 fates

4 major substances
can lead to stone
formation in the kidneys

**calcium
oxalate
stones**

**ammonium magnesium
phosphate stones**

**uric acid
stones**

**cystine
stones**

radiopaque on x-ray

radiopaque on x-ray

radiolucent on x-ray

caused by
genetic defect
which prevents
reabsorption
of cystine

most common =
70 - 80%

caused by chronic
urinary tract infections
with urease splitting
organisms including:
• *Proteus*
• *Klebsiella*

causes include:
• gout (see map)
• high purine diet
• myeloproliferative disease
• tumor lysis syndrome

2 subtypes:
• pure calcium oxalate
• mixed calcium oxalate
and phosphate

can lead to formation of
staghorn calculi

causes include:
• RTA
• sarcoid (see map)
• malignancy
• thyrotoxicosis (see map)
• low urinary citrate
• primary hyperparathyroidism (see map)
• idiopathic hypercalcuria
• hyperoxaluria
• high protein diet

obstruction

enter
ureter

pass through
urinary system
without obstructing
or causing pain

blocks outflow
of urine leading
to **hydronephrosis**

clinical presentation:
• severe pain
• hematuria
• frequency
• urgency
• dysuria

Fluid and Electrolyte Disorders

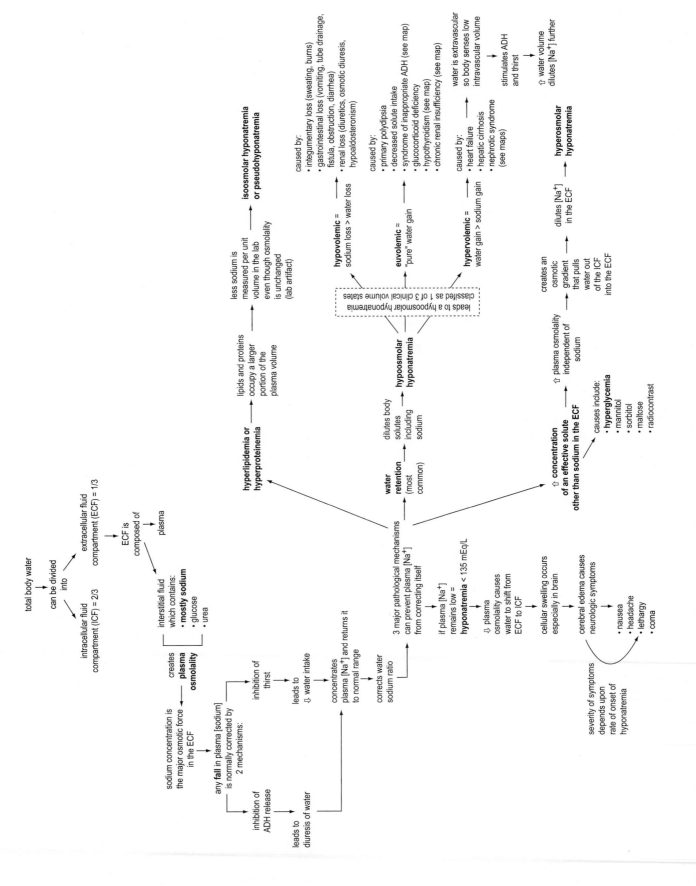

total body water

can be divided into

intracellular fluid compartment (ICF) = 2/3

extracellular fluid compartment (ECF) = 1/3

ECF is composed of

plasma

interstitial fluid which contains:
• mostly sodium
• glucose
• urea

creates plasma osmolality

sodium concentration is the major osmotic force in the ECF

any **fall** in plasma [sodium] is normally corrected by 2 mechanisms:

inhibition of thirst

inhibition of ADH release

leads to diuresis of water

leads to ⇓ water intake

concentrates plasma [Na⁺] and returns it to normal range

corrects water sodium ratio

3 major pathological mechanisms can prevent plasma [Na⁺] from correcting itself

if plasma [Na⁺] remains low = **hyponatremia** < 135 mEq/L

⇓ plasma osmolality causes water to shift from ECF to ICF

cellular swelling occurs especially in brain

cerebral edema causes neurologic symptoms

• nausea
• headache
• lethargy
• coma

severity of symptoms depends upon rate of onset of hyponatremia

hyperlipidemia or hyperproteinemia

lipids and proteins occupy a larger portion of the plasma volume

less sodium is measured per unit volume in the lab even though osmolality is unchanged (lab artifact)

isoosmolar hyponatremia or pseudohyponatremia

water retention (most common)

dilutes body solutes including sodium

hypoosmolar hyponatremia

leads to a hypoosmolar hyponatremia classified as 1 of 3 clinical volume states

hypovolemic = sodium loss > water loss

caused by:
• integumentary loss (sweating, burns)
• gastrointestinal loss (vomiting, tube drainage, fistula, obstruction, diarrhea)
• renal loss (diuretics, osmotic diuresis, hypoaldosteronism)

euvolemic = "pure" water gain

caused by:
• primary polydipsia
• decreased solute intake
• syndrome of inappropriate ADH (see map)
• glucocorticoid deficiency
• hypothyroidism (see map)
• chronic renal insufficiency (see map)

hypervolemic = water gain > sodium gain

caused by:
• heart failure
• hepatic cirrhosis
• nephrotic syndrome (see maps)

water is extravascular so body senses low intravascular volume

stimulates ADH and thirst

⇑ water volume dilutes [Na⁺] further

⇑ concentration of an effective solute other than sodium in the ECF

creates an osmotic gradient that pulls water out of the ICF into the ECF

dilutes [Na⁺] in the ECF

hyperosmolar hyponatremia

⇑ plasma osmolality independent of sodium

causes include:
• **hyperglycemia**
• mannitol
• sorbitol
• maltose
• radiocontrast

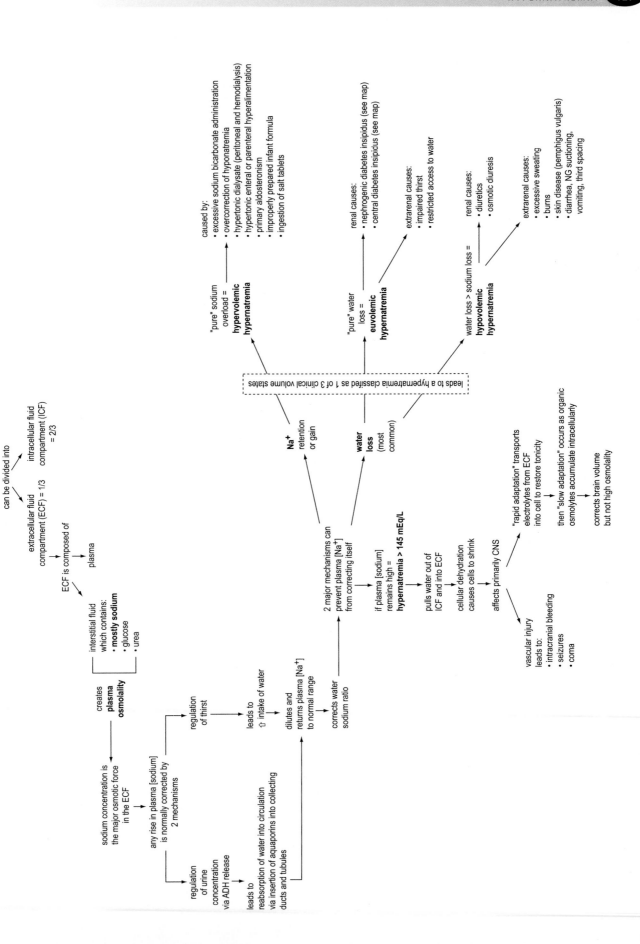

total body water

can be divided into

extracellular fluid compartment (ECF) = 1/3

intracellular fluid compartment (ICF) = 2/3

ECF is composed of

plasma

interstitial fluid which contains:
• **mostly sodium**
• glucose
• urea

creates **plasma osmolality**

sodium concentration is the major osmotic force in the ECF

any rise in plasma [sodium] is normally corrected by 2 mechanisms

regulation of thirst

leads to ⇧ intake of water

dilutes and returns plasma [Na⁺] to normal range

corrects water sodium ratio

regulation of urine concentration via ADH release

leads to reabsorption of water into circulation via insertion of aquaporins into collecting ducts and tubules

2 major mechanisms can prevent plasma [Na⁺] from correcting itself

Na⁺ retention or gain

water loss (most common)

leads to a hypernatremia classified as 1 of 3 clinical volume states

"pure" sodium overload = **hypervolemic hypernatremia**

caused by:
• excessive sodium bicarbonate administration
• overcorrection of hyponatremia
• hypertonic dialysate (peritoneal and hemodialysis)
• hypertonic enteral or parenteral hyperalimentation
• primary aldosteronism
• improperly prepared infant formula
• ingestion of salt tablets

"pure" water loss = **euvolemic hypernatremia**

renal causes:
• nephrogenic diabetes insipidus (see map)
• central diabetes insipidus (see map)

extrarenal causes:
• impaired thirst
• restricted access to water

water loss > sodium loss = **hypovolemic hypernatremia**

renal causes:
• diuretics
• osmotic diuresis

extrarenal causes:
• excessive sweating
• burns
• skin disease (pemphigus vulgaris)
• diarrhea, NG suctioning, vomiting, third spacing

if plasma [sodium] remains high = **hypernatremia > 145 mEq/L**

pulls water out of ICF and into ECF

cellular dehydration causes cells to shrink

affects primarily CNS

vascular injury leads to:
• intracranial bleeding
• seizures
• coma

"rapid adaptation" transports electrolytes from ECF into cell to restore tonicity

then "slow adaptation" occurs as organic osmolytes accumulate intracellularly

corrects brain volume but not high osmolality

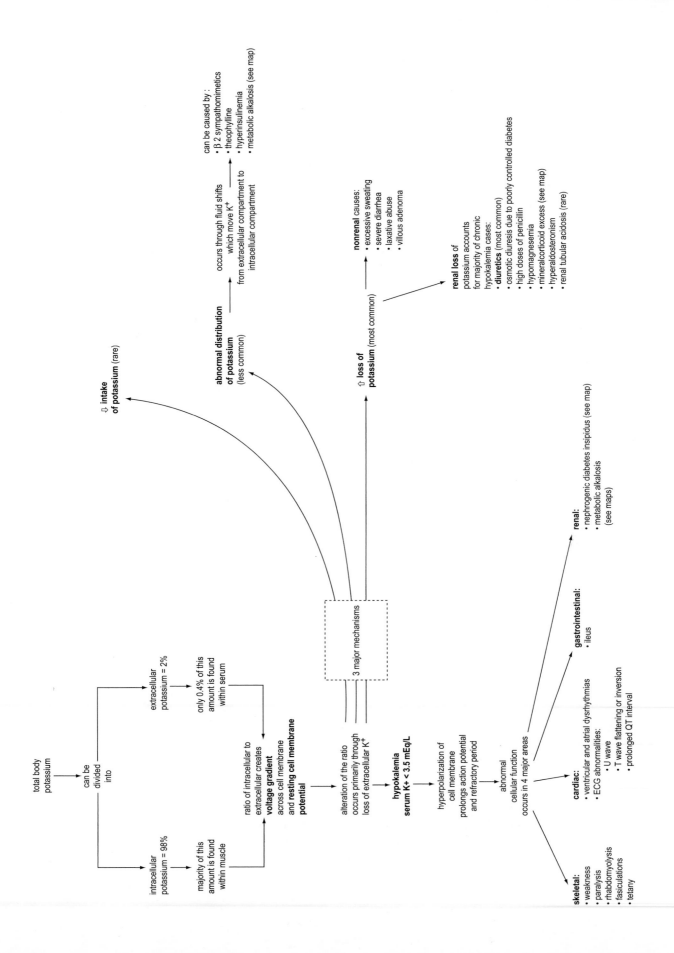

total body potassium
can be divided into

intracellular potassium = 98%
majority of this amount is found within muscle

extracellular potassium = 2%
only 0.4% of this amount is found within serum

ratio of intracellular to extracellular creates **voltage gradient** across cell membrane and **resting cell membrane potential**

3 major mechanisms

⇩ **intake of potassium** (rare)

abnormal distribution of potassium (less common)
occurs through fluid shifts which move K⁺ from extracellular compartment to intracellular compartment

can be caused by:
• β 2 sympathomimetics
• theophylline
• hyperinsulinemia
• metabolic alkalosis (see map)

⇧ **loss of potassium** (most common)

nonrenal causes:
• excessive sweating
• severe diarrhea
• laxative abuse
• villous adenoma

renal loss of potassium accounts for majority of chronic hypokalemia cases:
• **diuretics** (most common)
• osmotic diuresis due to poorly controlled diabetes
• high doses of penicillin
• hypomagnesemia
• mineralcorticoid excess (see map)
• hyperaldosteronism
• renal tubular acidosis (rare)

alteration of the ratio occurs primarily through loss of extracellular K⁺

hypokalemia serum K+ < 3.5 mEq/L

hyperpolarization of cell membrane prolongs action potential and refractory period

abnormal cellular function occurs in 4 major areas

skeletal:
• weakness
• paralysis
• rhabdomyolysis
• fasciculations
• tetany

cardiac:
• ventricular and atrial dysrhythmias
• ECG abnormalities:
 • U wave
 • T wave flattening or inversion
 • prolonged QT interval

gastrointestinal:
• ileus

renal:
• nephrogenic diabetes insipidus (see map)
• metabolic alkalosis (see maps)

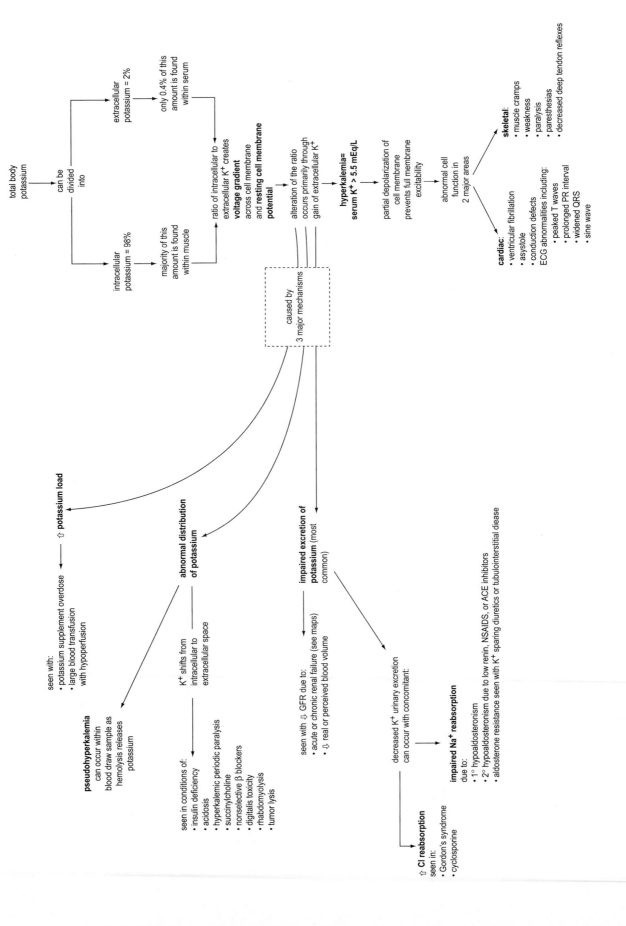

total body potassium

can be divided into

intracellular potassium = 98%

extracellular potassium = 2%

majority of this amount is found within muscle

only 0.4% of this amount is found within serum

ratio of intracellular to extracellular K⁺ creates **voltage gradient** across cell membrane and **resting cell membrane potential**

alteration of the ratio occurs primarily through gain of extracellular K⁺

hyperkalemia= serum K⁺ > 5.5 mEq/L

partial depolarization of cell membrane prevents full membrane excitability

abnormal cell function in 2 major areas

skeletal:
• muscle cramps
• weakness
• paralysis
• paresthesias
• decreased deep tendon reflexes

cardiac:
• ventricular fibrillation
• asystole
• conduction defects
ECG abnormalities including:
• peaked T waves
• prolonged PR interval
• widened QRS
• sine wave

caused by 3 major mechanisms

seen with:
• potassium supplement overdose
• large blood transfusion with hypoperfusion

⇧ **potassium load**

abnormal distribution of potassium

impaired excretion of potassium (most common)

pseudohyperkalemia
can occur within blood draw sample as hemolysis releases potassium

K⁺ shifts from intracellular to extracellular space

seen in conditions of:
• insulin deficiency
• acidosis
• hyperkalemic periodic paralysis
• succinylcholine
• nonselective β blockers
• digitalis toxicity
• rhabdomyolysis
• tumor lysis

seen with ⇩ GFR due to:
• acute or chronic renal failure (see maps)
• ⇩ real or perceived blood volume

decreased K⁺ urinary excretion can occur with concomitant:

impaired Na⁺ reabsorption
due to:
• 1° hypoaldosteronism
• 2° hypoaldosteronism due to low renin, NSAIDS, or ACE inhibitors
• aldosterone resistance seen with K⁺ sparing diuretics or tubulointerstitial diease

⇧ **Cl reabsorption**
seen in:
• Gordon's syndrome
• cyclosporine

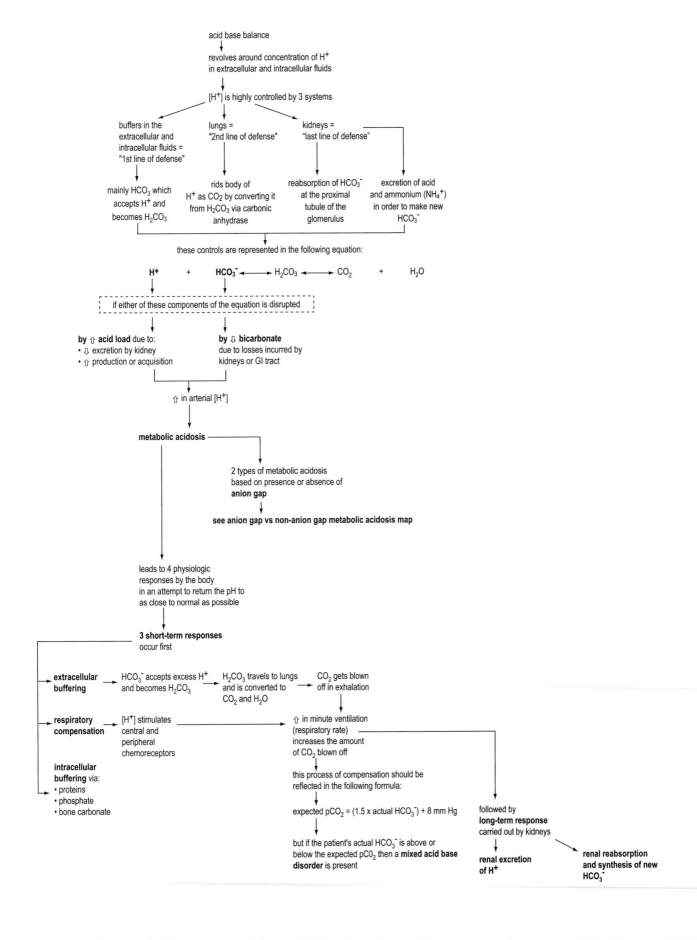

acid base balance

revolves around concentration of H^+
in extracellular and intracellular fluids

[H^+] is highly controlled by 3 systems

buffers in the
extracellular and
intracellular fluids =
"1st line of defense"

lungs =
"2nd line of defense"

kidneys =
"last line of defense"

mainly HCO_3 which
accepts H^+ and
becomes H_2CO_3

rids body of
H^+ as CO_2 by converting it
from H_2CO_3 via carbonic
anhydrase

reabsorption of HCO_3^-
at the proximal
tubule of the
glomerulus

excretion of acid
and ammonium (NH_4^+)
in order to make new
HCO_3^-

these controls are represented in the following equation:

$$H^+ \quad + \quad HCO_3^- \longleftrightarrow H_2CO_3 \longleftrightarrow CO_2 \quad + \quad H_2O$$

if either of these components of the equation is disrupted

by ⇧ **acid load** due to:
• ⇩ excretion by kidney
• ⇧ production or acquisition

by ⇩ **bicarbonate**
due to losses incurred by
kidneys or GI tract

⇧ in arterial [H^+]

metabolic acidosis

2 types of metabolic acidosis
based on presence or absence of
anion gap

see anion gap vs non-anion gap metabolic acidosis map

leads to 4 physiologic
responses by the body
in an attempt to return the pH to
as close to normal as possible

3 short-term responses
occur first

**extracellular
buffering**

HCO_3^- accepts excess H^+
and becomes H_2CO_3

H_2CO_3 travels to lungs
and is converted to
CO_2 and H_2O

CO_2 gets blown
off in exhalation

**respiratory
compensation**

[H^+] stimulates
central and
peripheral
chemoreceptors

⇧ in minute ventilation
(respiratory rate)
increases the amount
of CO_2 blown off

this process of compensation should be
reflected in the following formula:

expected pCO_2 = (1.5 x actual HCO_3^-) + 8 mm Hg

but if the patient's actual HCO_3^- is above or
below the expected pCO_2 then a **mixed acid base
disorder** is present

**intracellular
buffering** via:
• proteins
• phosphate
• bone carbonate

followed by
long-term response
carried out by kidneys

**renal excretion
of H^+**

**renal reabsorption
and synthesis of new
HCO_3^-**

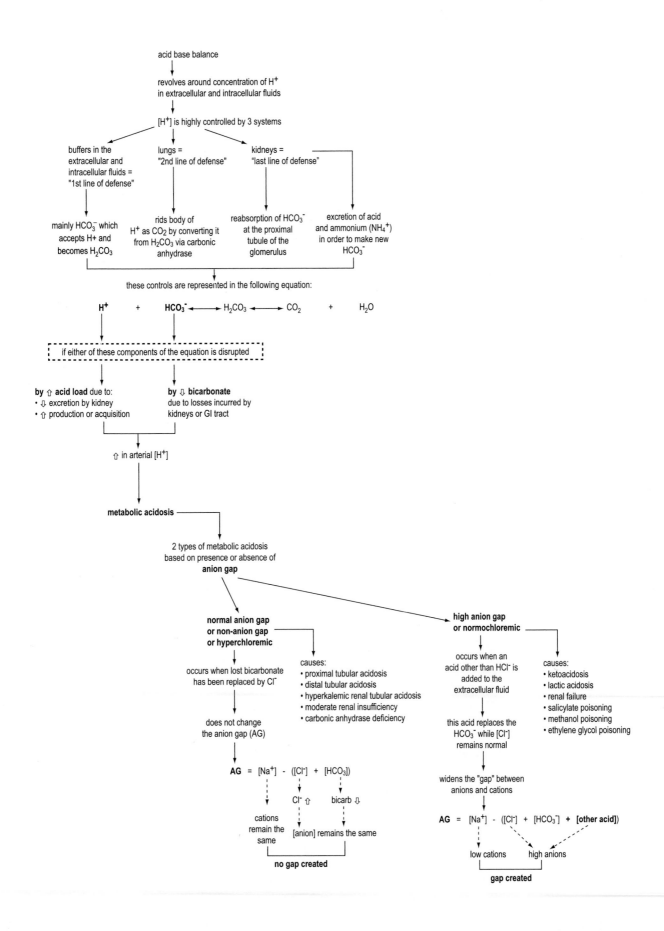

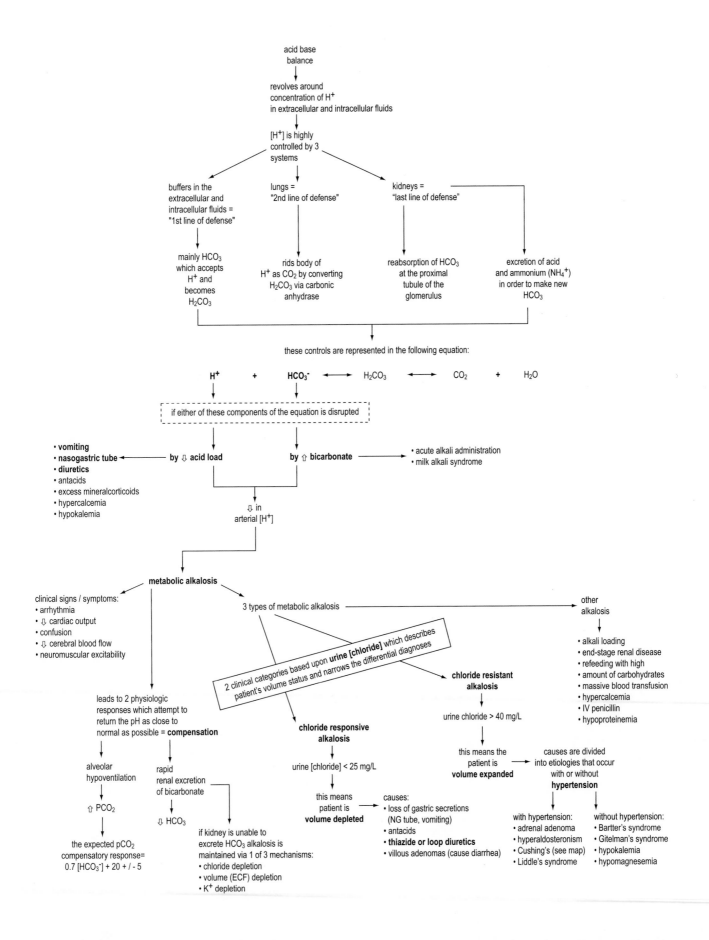

acid base balance

↓

revolves around concentration of H⁺ in extracellular and intracellular fluids

↓

[H⁺] is highly controlled by 3 systems

buffers in the extracellular and intracellular fluids = "1st line of defense"

lungs = "2nd line of defense"

kidneys = "last line of defense"

mainly HCO₃ which accepts H⁺ and becomes H₂CO₃

rids body of H⁺ as CO₂ by converting H₂CO₃ via carbonic anhydrase

reabsorption of HCO₃ at the proximal tubule of the glomerulus

excretion of acid and ammonium (NH₄⁺) in order to make new HCO₃

these controls are represented in the following equation:

$$H^+ \; + \; HCO_3^- \longleftrightarrow H_2CO_3 \longleftrightarrow CO_2 \; + \; H_2O$$

if either of these components of the equation is disrupted

by ⇩ acid load

- **vomiting**
- **nasogastric tube**
- **diuretics**
- antacids
- excess mineralcorticoids
- hypercalcemia
- hypokalemia

by ⇧ bicarbonate

- acute alkali administration
- milk alkali syndrome

⇩ in arterial [H⁺]

metabolic alkalosis

clinical signs / symptoms:
- arrhythmia
- ⇩ cardiac output
- confusion
- ⇩ cerebral blood flow
- neuromuscular excitability

3 types of metabolic alkalosis

other alkalosis

2 clinical categories based upon **urine [chloride]** which describes patient's volume status and narrows the differential diagnoses

- alkali loading
- end-stage renal disease
- refeeding with high amount of carbohydrates
- massive blood transfusion
- hypercalcemia
- IV penicillin
- hypoproteinemia

leads to 2 physiologic responses which attempt to return the pH as close to normal as possible = **compensation**

chloride resistant alkalosis

urine chloride > 40 mg/L

chloride responsive alkalosis

alveolar hypoventilation

rapid renal excretion of bicarbonate

urine [chloride] < 25 mg/L

this means the patient is **volume expanded**

causes are divided into etiologies that occur with or without **hypertension**

⇧ PCO₂

⇩ HCO₃

this means patient is **volume depleted**

the expected pCO₂ compensatory response= 0.7 [HCO₃⁻] + 20 + / - 5

if kidney is unable to excrete HCO₃ alkalosis is maintained via 1 of 3 mechanisms:
- chloride depletion
- volume (ECF) depletion
- K⁺ depletion

causes:
- loss of gastric secretions (NG tube, vomiting)
- antacids
- **thiazide or loop diuretics**
- villous adenomas (cause diarrhea)

with hypertension:
- adrenal adenoma
- hyperaldosteronism
- Cushing's (see map)
- Liddle's syndrome

without hypertension:
- Bartter's syndrome
- Gitelman's syndrome
- hypokalemia
- hypomagnesemia

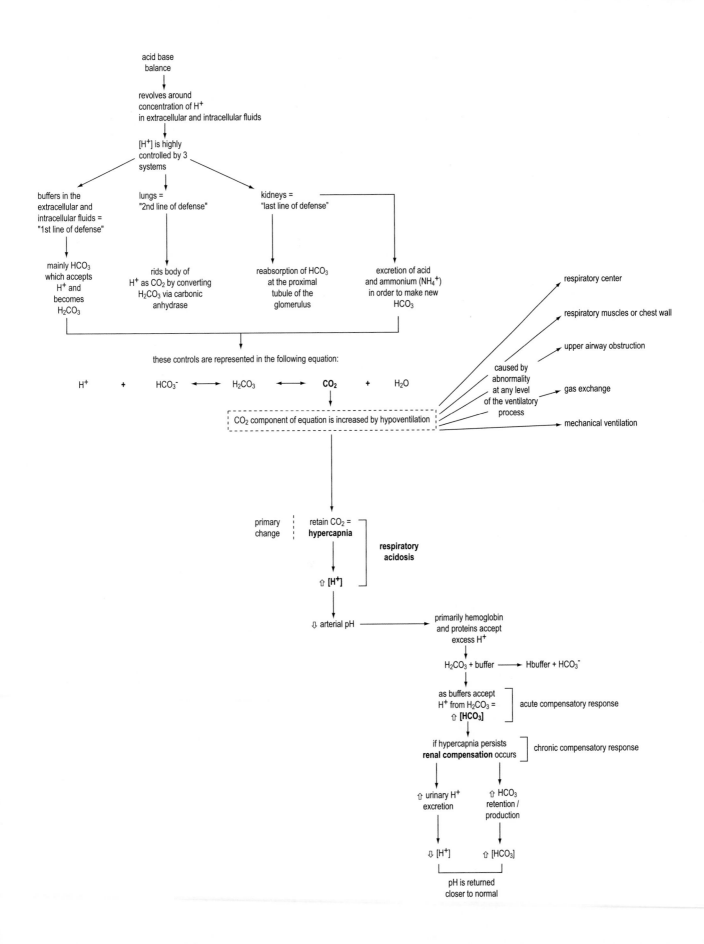

acid base balance

revolves around concentration of H$^+$ in extracellular and intracellular fluids

[H$^+$] is highly controlled by 3 systems

buffers in the extracellular and intracellular fluids = "1st line of defense"

lungs = "2nd line of defense"

kidneys = "last line of defense"

mainly HCO$_3$ which accepts H$^+$ and becomes H$_2$CO$_3$

rids body of H$^+$ as CO$_2$ by converting H$_2$CO$_3$ via carbonic anhydrase

reabsorption of HCO$_3$ at the proximal tubule of the glomerulus

excretion of acid and ammonium (NH$_4^+$) in order to make new HCO$_3$

these controls are represented in the following equation:

$$H^+ \quad + \quad HCO_3^- \quad \longleftrightarrow \quad H_2CO_3 \quad \longleftrightarrow \quad CO_2 \quad + \quad H_2O$$

CO$_2$ component of equation is increased by hypoventilation

caused by abnormality at any level of the ventilatory process

respiratory center

respiratory muscles or chest wall

upper airway obstruction

gas exchange

mechanical ventilation

primary change

retain CO$_2$ = **hypercapnia**

respiratory acidosis

⇧ [H$^+$]

⇩ arterial pH

primarily hemoglobin and proteins accept excess H$^+$

H$_2$CO$_3$ + buffer ⟶ Hbuffer + HCO$_3^-$

as buffers accept H$^+$ from H$_2$CO$_3$ = ⇧ [HCO$_3$]

acute compensatory response

if hypercapnia persists **renal compensation** occurs

chronic compensatory response

⇧ urinary H$^+$ excretion

⇧ HCO$_3$ retention / production

⇩ [H$^+$]

⇧ [HCO$_3$]

pH is returned closer to normal

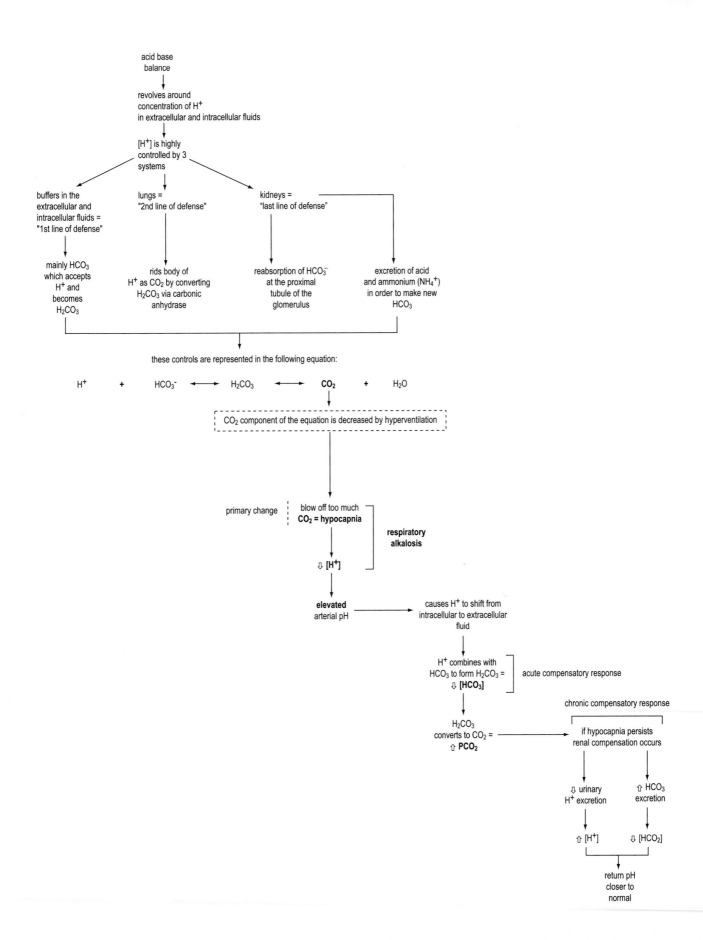

Immune Mediated Disorders

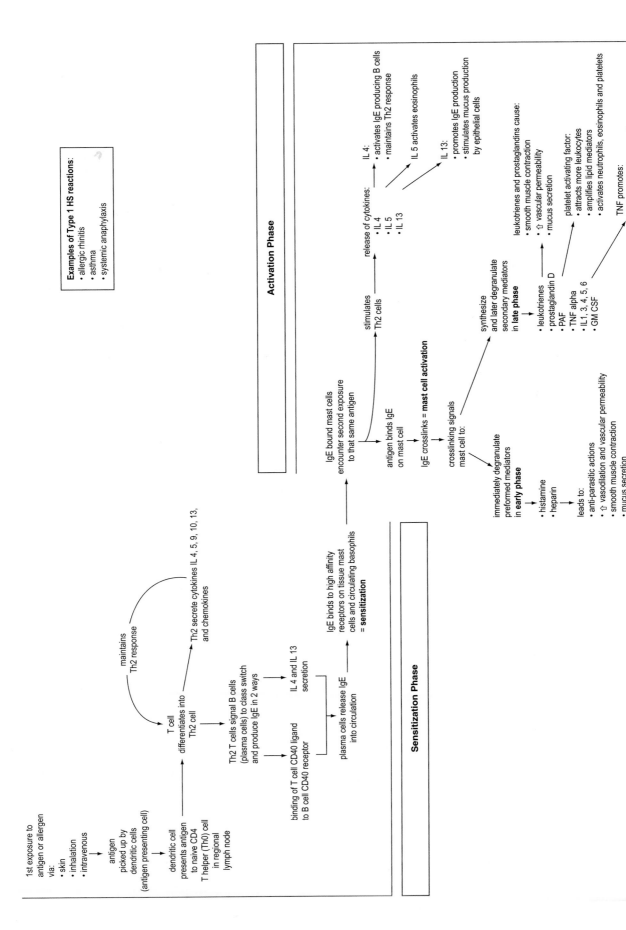

Examples of Type 1 HS reactions:
• allergic rhinitis
• asthma
• systemic anaphylaxis

Activation Phase

IgE bound mast cells encounter second exposure to that same antigen

antigen binds IgE on mast cell

IgE crosslinks = **mast cell activation**

crosslinking signals mast cell to:

immediately degranulate preformed mediators in **early phase**
• histamine
• heparin

leads to:
• anti-parasitic actions
• ⇧ vasodilation and vascular permeability
• smooth muscle contraction
• mucus secretion

synthesize and later degranulate secondary mediators in **late phase**
• leukotrienes
• prostaglandin D
• PAF
• TNF alpha
• IL1, 3, 4, 5, 6
• GM CSF

leukotrienes and prostaglandins cause:
• smooth muscle contraction
• ⇧ vascular permeability
• mucus secretion

platelet activating factor:
• attracts more leukocytes
• amplifies lipid mediators
• activates neutrophils, eosinophils and platelets

TNF promotes:
• inflammation (see maps)
• cytokine production
• activation of endothelium

stimulates Th2 cells

release of cytokines:
• IL 4
• IL 5
• IL 13

IL 4:
• activates IgE producing B cells
• maintains Th2 response

IL 5 activates eosinophils

IL 13:
• promotes IgE production
• stimulates mucus production by epithelial cells

Sensitization Phase

1st exposure to antigen or allergen via:
• skin
• inhalation
• intravenous

antigen picked up by dendritic cells (antigen presenting cell)

dendritic cell presents antigen to naive CD4 T helper (Th0) cell in regional lymph node

T cell differentiates into Th2 cell

maintains Th2 response

Th2 secrete cytokines IL 4, 5, 9, 10, 13, and chemokines

Th2 T cells (plasma cells) signal B cells to class switch and produce IgE in 2 ways

binding of T cell CD40 ligand to B cell CD40 receptor

IL 4 and IL 13 secretion

plasma cells release IgE into circulation

IgE binds to high affinity receptors on tissue mast cells and circulating basophils = **sensitization**

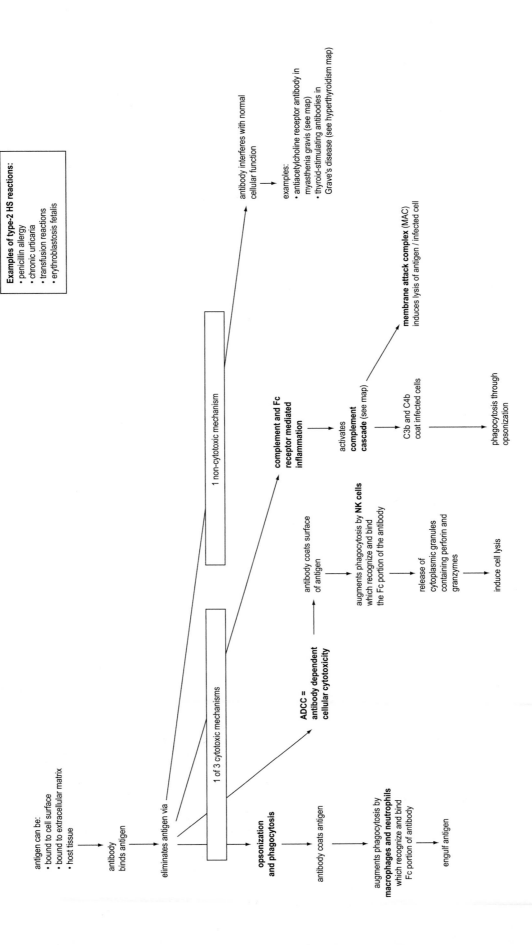

Examples of type-2 HS reactions:
- penicillin allergy
- chronic urticaria
- transfusion reactions
- erythroblastosis fetalis

antigen can be:
- bound to cell surface
- bound to extracellular matrix
- host tissue

antibody binds antigen → eliminates antigen via

1 non-cytotoxic mechanism

antibody interferes with normal cellular function

examples:
- antiacetylcholine receptor antibody in myasthenia gravis (see map)
- thyroid-stimulating antibodies in Grave's disease (see hyperthyroidism map)

complement and Fc receptor mediated inflammation → activates **complement cascade** (see map) → C3b and C4b coat infected cells → phagocytosis through opsonization

membrane attack complex (MAC)
induces lysis of antigen / infected cell

1 of 3 cytotoxic mechanisms

ADCC = antibody dependent cellular cytotoxicity → antibody coats surface of antigen → augments phagocytosis by **NK cells** which recognize and bind the Fc portion of the antibody → release of cytoplasmic granules containing perforin and granzymes → induce cell lysis

opsonization and phagocytosis → antibody coats antigen → augments phagocytosis by **macrophages and neutrophils** which recognize and bind Fc portion of antibody → engulf antigen

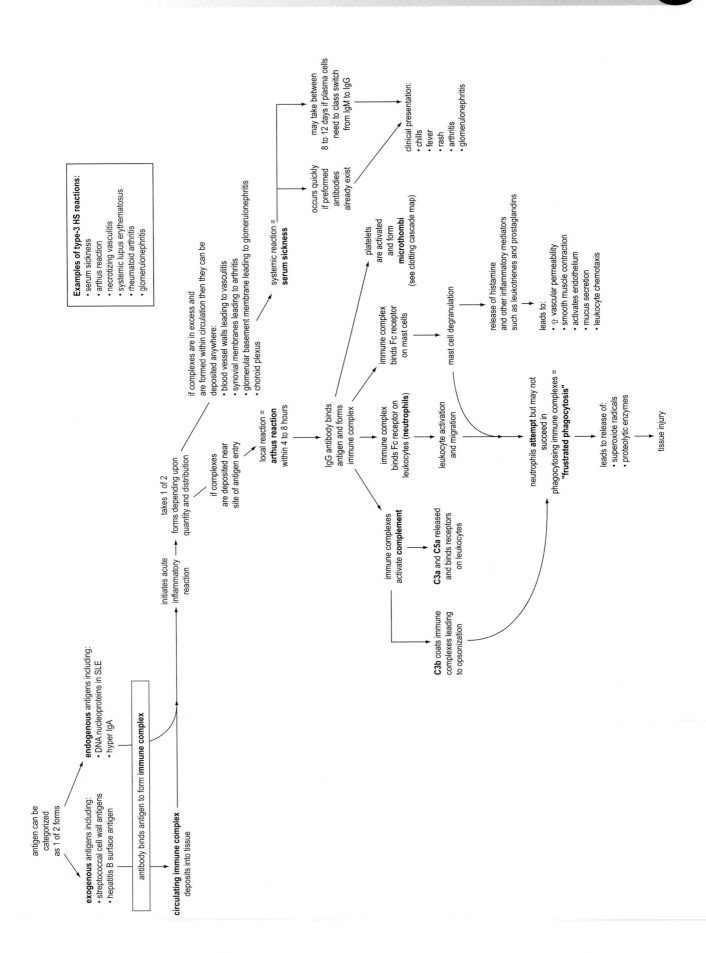

antigen can be categorized as 1 of 2 forms

exogenous antigens including:
• streptococcal cell wall antigens
• hepatitis B surface antigen

endogenous antigens including:
• DNA nucleoproteins in SLE
• hyper IgA

antibody binds antigen to form **immune complex**

circulating immune complex deposits into tissue

initiates acute inflammatory reaction

takes 1 of 2 forms depending upon quantity and distribution

if complexes are in excess and are formed within circulation then they can be deposited anywhere:
• blood vessel walls leading to vasculitis
• synovial membranes leading to arthritis
• glomerular basement membrane leading to glomerulonephritis
• choroid plexus

systemic reaction = **serum sickness**

occurs quickly if preformed antibodies already exist

may take between 8 to 12 days if plasma cells need to class switch from IgM to IgG

clinical presentation:
• chills
• fever
• rash
• arthritis
• glomerulonephritis

if complexes are deposited near site of antigen entry

local reaction = **arthus reaction** within 4 to 8 hours

IgG antibody binds antigen and forms immune complex

immune complex binds Fc receptor on mast cells

mast cell degranulation

release of histamine and other inflammatory mediators such as leukotrienes and prostaglandins

leads to:
• ⇧ vascular permeability
• smooth muscle contraction
• activates endothelium
• mucus secretion
• leukocyte chemotaxis

platelets are activated and form **microthombi** (see clotting cascade map)

immune complex binds Fc receptor on leukocytes (**neutrophils**)

leukocyte activation and migration

neutrophils **attempt** but may not succeed in phagocytosing immune complexes = **"frustrated phagocytosis"**

leads to release of:
• superoxide radicals
• proteolytic enzymes

tissue injury

immune complexes activate **complement**

C3a and **C5a** released and binds receptors on leukocytes

C3b coats immune complexes leading to opsonization

Examples of type-3 HS reactions:
• serum sickness
• arthus reaction
• necrotizing vasculitis
• systemic lupus erythematosus
• rheumatoid arthritis
• glomerulonephritis

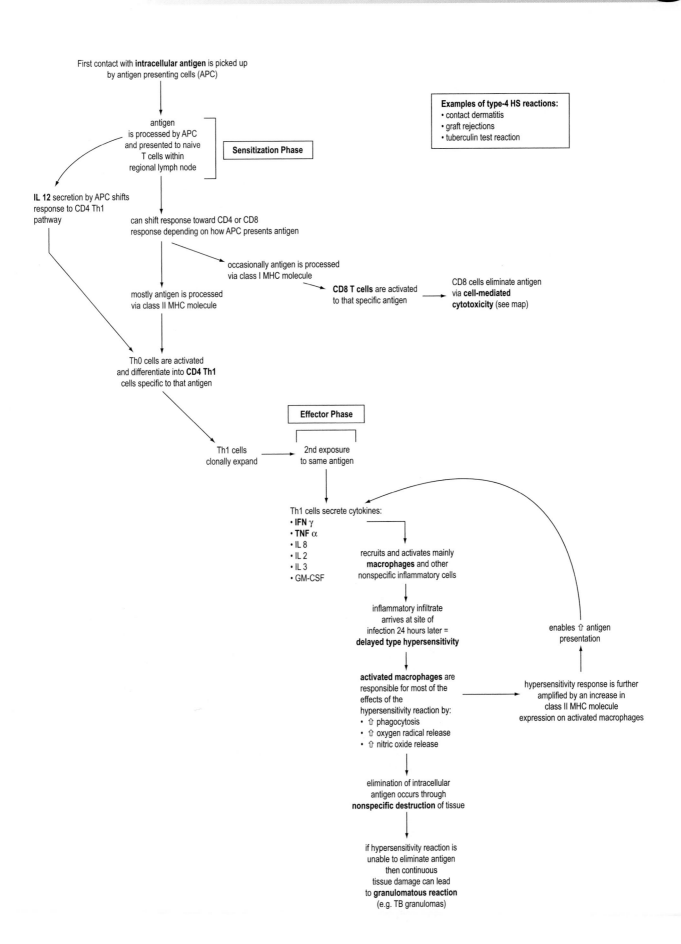

First contact with **intracellular antigen** is picked up
by antigen presenting cells (APC)

antigen
is processed by APC
and presented to naive
T cells within
regional lymph node

Sensitization Phase

Examples of type-4 HS reactions:
• contact dermatitis
• graft rejections
• tuberculin test reaction

IL 12 secretion by APC shifts
response to CD4 Th1
pathway

can shift response toward CD4 or CD8
response depending on how APC presents antigen

occasionally antigen is processed
via class I MHC molecule

mostly antigen is processed
via class II MHC molecule

CD8 T cells are activated
to that specific antigen

CD8 cells eliminate antigen
via **cell-mediated
cytotoxicity** (see map)

Th0 cells are activated
and differentiate into **CD4 Th1**
cells specific to that antigen

Effector Phase

Th1 cells
clonally expand

2nd exposure
to same antigen

Th1 cells secrete cytokines:
• **IFN** γ
• **TNF** α
• IL 8
• IL 2
• IL 3
• GM-CSF

recruits and activates mainly
macrophages and other
nonspecific inflammatory cells

inflammatory infiltrate
arrives at site of
infection 24 hours later =
delayed type hypersensitivity

enables ⇧ antigen
presentation

activated macrophages are
responsible for most of the
effects of the
hypersensitivity reaction by:
• ⇧ phagocytosis
• ⇧ oxygen radical release
• ⇧ nitric oxide release

hypersensitivity response is further
amplified by an increase in
class II MHC molecule
expression on activated macrophages

elimination of intracellular
antigen occurs through
nonspecific destruction of tissue

if hypersensitivity reaction is
unable to eliminate antigen
then continuous
tissue damage can lead
to **granulomatous reaction**
(e.g. TB granulomas)

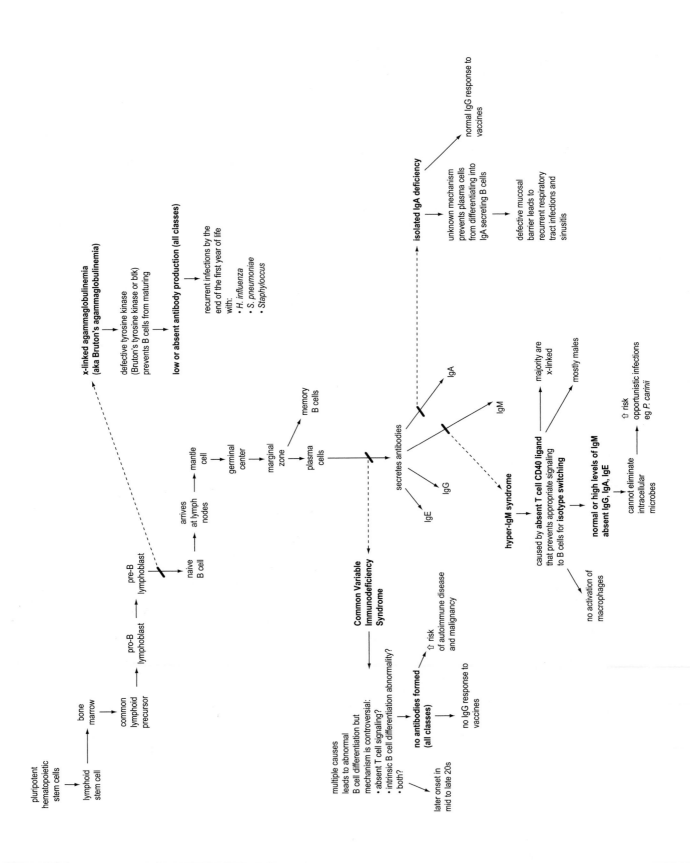

pluripotent hematopoietic stem cells

lymphoid stem cell

bone marrow

common lymphoid precursor

pro-B lymphoblast

pre-B lymphoblast

naive B cell

arrives at lymph nodes

mantle cell

germinal center

marginal zone

plasma cells

memory B cells

secretes antibodies

IgA

IgM

IgG

IgE

x-linked agammaglobulinemia (aka Bruton's agammaglobulinemia)

defective tyrosine kinase (Bruton's tyrosine kinase or btk) prevents B cells from maturing

low or absent antibody production (all classes)

recurrent infections by the end of the first year of life with:
- *H. influenza*
- *S. pneumoniae*
- *Staphyloccus*

isolated IgA deficiency

normal IgG response to vaccines

unknown mechanism prevents plasma cells from differentiating into IgA secreting B cells

defective mucosal barrier leads to recurrent respiratory tract infections and sinusitis

hyper-IgM syndrome

caused by **absent T cell CD40 ligand** that prevents appropriate signaling to B cells for **isotype switching**

majority are x-linked

mostly males

normal or high levels of IgM absent IgG, IgA, IgE

cannot eliminate intracellular microbes

⇧ risk opportunistic infections eg *P. carnii*

no activation of macrophages

Common Variable Immunodeficiency Syndrome

multiple causes leads to abnormal B cell differentiation but mechanism is controversial:
- absent T cell signaling?
- intrinsic B cell differentiation abnormality?
- both?

later onset in mid to late 20s

no antibodies formed (all classes)

⇧ risk of autoimmune disease and malignancy

no IgG response to vaccines

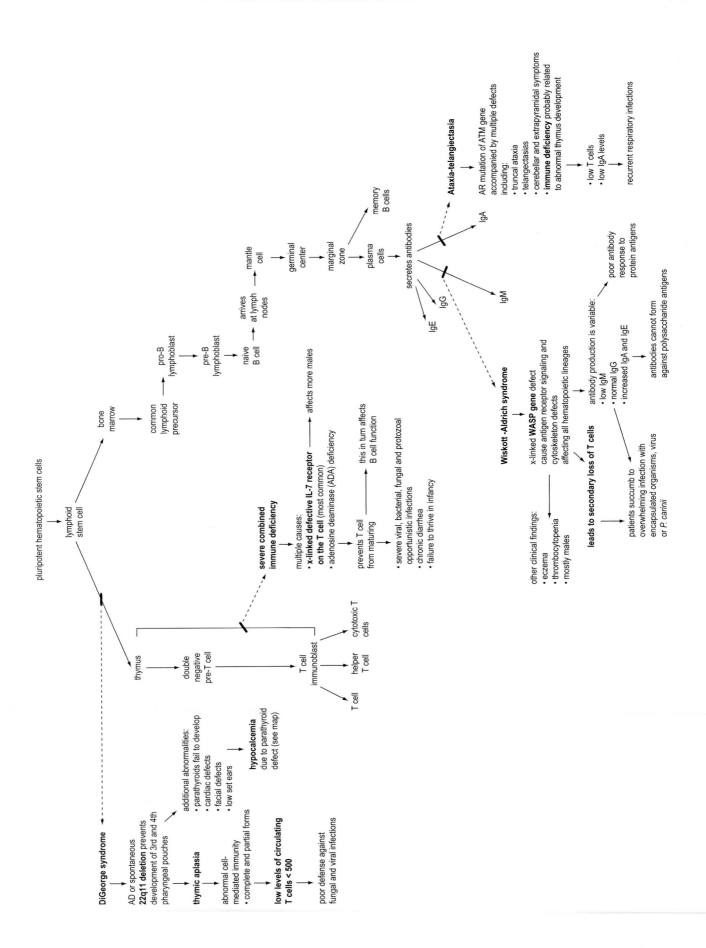

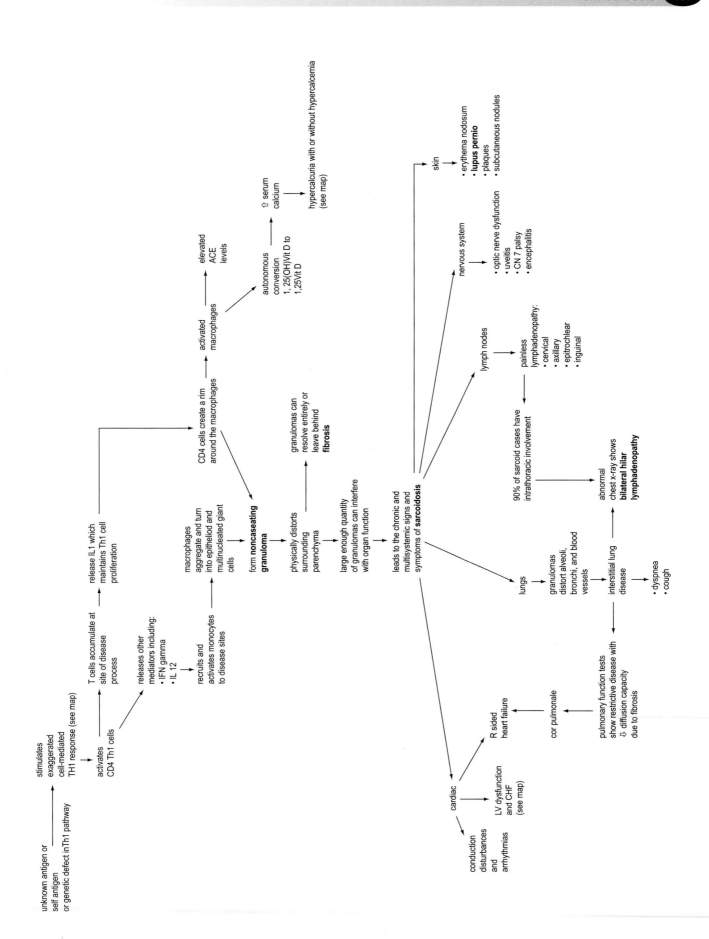

unknown antigen or self antigen or genetic defect in Th1 pathway

stimulates exaggerated cell-mediated TH1 response (see map)

activates CD4 Th1 cells

T cells accumulate at site of disease process → release IL1 which maintains Th1 cell proliferation

releases other mediators including:
• IFN gamma
• IL 12

recruits and activates monocytes to disease sites

macrophages aggregate and turn into epitheliod and multinucleated giant cells

form **noncaseating granuloma**

CD4 cells create a rim around the macrophages

activated macrophages → elevated ACE levels

autonomous conversion 1, 25(OH)Vit D to 1,25Vit D

⇧ serum calcium → hypercalcuria with or without hypercalcemia (see map)

granulomas can resolve entirely or leave behind **fibrosis**

physically distorts surrounding parenchyma

large enough quantity of granulomas can interfere with organ function

leads to the chronic and multisystemic signs and symptoms of **sarcoidosis**

skin
• erythema nodosum
• **lupus pernio**
• plaques
• subcutaneous nodules

nervous system
• optic nerve dysfunction
• uveitis
• CN 7 palsy
• encephalitis

lymph nodes → painless lymphadenopathy:
• cervical
• axillary
• epitrochlear
• inguinal

90% of sarcoid cases have intrathoracic involvement

abnormal chest x-ray shows **bilateral hilar lymphadenopathy**

lungs → granulomas distort alveoli, bronchi, and blood vessels → interstitial lung disease → • dyspnea • cough

pulmonary function tests show restrictive disease with ⇩ diffusion capacity due to fibrosis → cor pulmonale → R sided heart failure

cardiac
• conduction disturbances and arrhythmias
• LV dysfunction and CHF (see map)

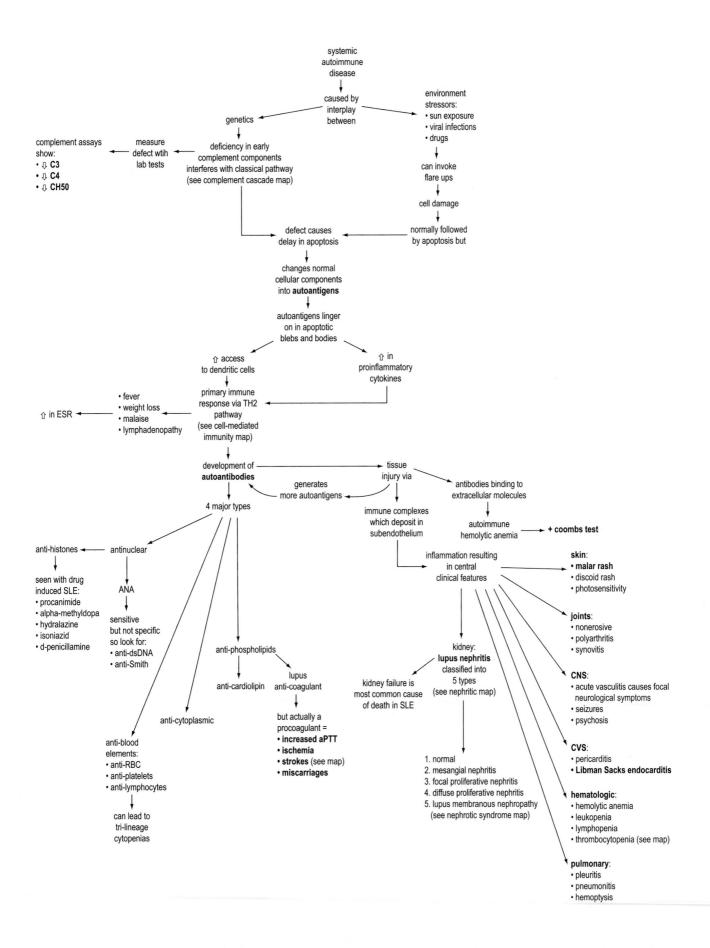

systemic
autoimmune
disease

caused by
interplay
between

environment
stressors:
• sun exposure
• viral infections
• drugs

genetics

complement assays
show:
• ⇩ C3
• ⇩ C4
• ⇩ CH50

measure
defect wtih
lab tests

deficiency in early
complement components
interferes with classical pathway
(see complement cascade map)

can invoke
flare ups

cell damage

normally followed
by apoptosis but

defect causes
delay in apoptosis

changes normal
cellular components
into **autoantigens**

autoantigens linger
on in apoptotic
blebs and bodies

⇧ access
to dendritic cells

⇧ in
proinflammatory
cytokines

• fever
• weight loss
• malaise
• lymphadenopathy

⇧ in ESR

primary immune
response via TH2
pathway
(see cell-mediated
immunity map)

development of
autoantibodies

generates
more autoantigens

tissue
injury via

antibodies binding to
extracellular molecules

immune complexes
which deposit in
subendothelium

autoimmune
hemolytic anemia

→ + coombs test

4 major types

anti-histones

antinuclear

seen with drug
induced SLE:
• procanimide
• alpha-methyldopa
• hydralazine
• isoniazid
• d-penicillamine

ANA

sensitive
but not specific
so look for:
• anti-dsDNA
• anti-Smith

anti-phospholipids

anti-cardiolipin

lupus
anti-coagulant

anti-cytoplasmic

but actually a
procoagulant =
• **increased aPTT**
• **ischemia**
• **strokes** (see map)
• **miscarriages**

anti-blood
elements:
• anti-RBC
• anti-platelets
• anti-lymphocytes

can lead to
tri-lineage
cytopenias

inflammation resulting
in central
clinical features

kidney failure is
most common cause
of death in SLE

kidney:
lupus nephritis
classified into
5 types
(see nephritic map)

1. normal
2. mesangial nephritis
3. focal proliferative nephritis
4. diffuse proliferative nephritis
5. lupus membranous nephropathy
   (see nephrotic syndrome map)

skin:
• **malar rash**
• discoid rash
• photosensitivity

joints:
• nonerosive
• polyarthritis
• synovitis

CNS:
• acute vasculitis causes focal
  neurological symptoms
• seizures
• psychosis

CVS:
• pericarditis
• **Libman Sacks endocarditis**

hematologic:
• hemolytic anemia
• leukopenia
• lymphopenia
• thrombocytopenia (see map)

pulmonary:
• pleuritis
• pneumonitis
• hemoptysis

Infectious Disorders

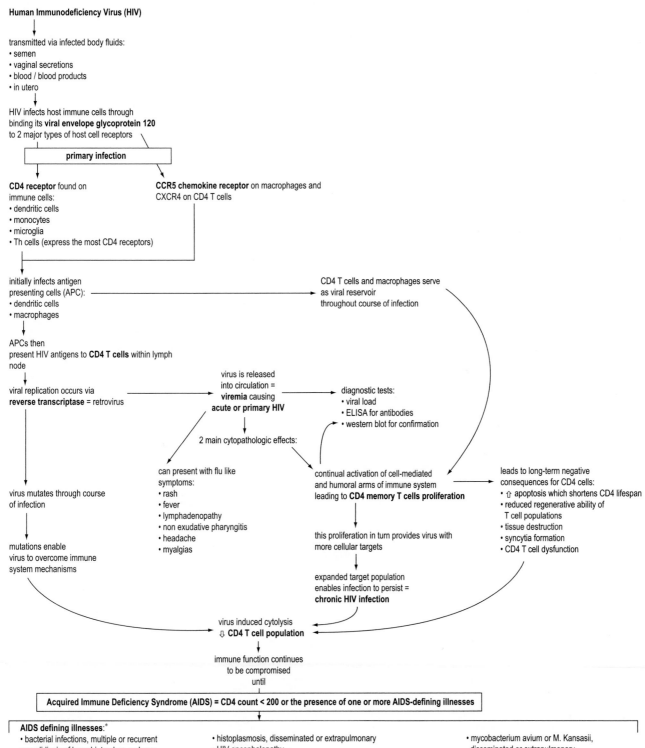

Human Immunodeficiency Virus (HIV)

transmitted via infected body fluids:
• semen
• vaginal secretions
• blood / blood products
• in utero

HIV infects host immune cells through
binding its **viral envelope glycoprotein 120**
to 2 major types of host cell receptors

primary infection

CD4 receptor found on
immune cells:
• dendritic cells
• monocytes
• microglia
• Th cells (express the most CD4 receptors)

CCR5 chemokine receptor on macrophages and
CXCR4 on CD4 T cells

initially infects antigen
presenting cells (APC):
• dendritic cells
• macrophages

CD4 T cells and macrophages serve
as viral reservoir
throughout course of infection

APCs then
present HIV antigens to **CD4 T cells** within lymph
node

viral replication occurs via
reverse transcriptase = retrovirus

virus is released
into circulation =
viremia causing
acute or primary HIV

diagnostic tests:
• viral load
• ELISA for antibodies
• western blot for confirmation

2 main cytopathologic effects:

can present with flu like
symptoms:
• rash
• fever
• lymphadenopathy
• non exudative pharyngitis
• headache
• myalgias

continual activation of cell-mediated
and humoral arms of immune system
leading to **CD4 memory T cells proliferation**

leads to long-term negative
consequences for CD4 cells:
• ⇧ apoptosis which shortens CD4 lifespan
• reduced regenerative ability of
  T cell populations
• tissue destruction
• syncytia formation
• CD4 T cell dysfunction

virus mutates through course
of infection

this proliferation in turn provides virus with
more cellular targets

mutations enable
virus to overcome immune
system mechanisms

expanded target population
enables infection to persist =
chronic HIV infection

virus induced cytolysis
⇩ **CD4 T cell population**

immune function continues
to be compromised
until

Acquired Immune Deficiency Syndrome (AIDS) = CD4 count < 200 or the presence of one or more AIDS-defining illnesses

AIDS defining illnesses:[*]
• bacterial infections, multiple or recurrent
• candidiasis of bronchi, trachea, or lungs
• candidiasis of esophagus
• carcinoma, invasive cervical
• coccidiodomycosis, disseminated or extrapulmonary
• cryptococcosis, extrapulmonary
• cryptosporidiosis, chronic intestinal
• cytomegalovirus disease (retinitis or other)
• herpes simplex, with esophagitis, pneumonitis, or
  chronic mucocutaneous ulcers

• histoplasmosis, disseminated or extrapulmonary
• HIV encephalopathy
• HIV wasting syndrome
• immunosuppression (severe HIV-related)
• isosporiasis, chronic intestinal
• Kaposi's sarcoma
• lymphoid interstitial pneumonia and/or pulmonary lymphoid hyperplasia
• lymphoma, Burkitt's
• lymphoma, immunoblastic
• lymphoma, primary in brain

• mycobacterium avium or M. Kansasii,
  disseminated or extrapulmonary
• M. tuberculosis, disseminated or extrampulmonary
• M. tuberculosis, pulmonary
• mycobacterial disease, other
• pneumocystis jiroveci pneumonia
• progressive multifocal leukoencephalopathy
• salmonella septicemia, recurrent
• toxoplasmosis of brain

[*]CDC's AIDS surveillance case definition conditions.

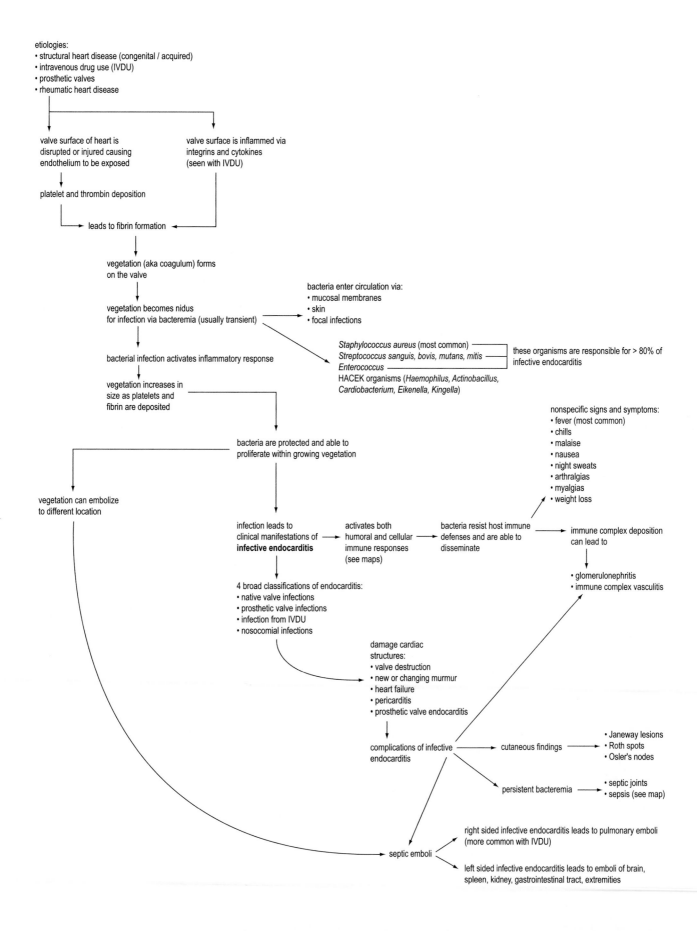

etiologies:
• structural heart disease (congenital / acquired)
• intravenous drug use (IVDU)
• prosthetic valves
• rheumatic heart disease

valve surface of heart is disrupted or injured causing endothelium to be exposed

valve surface is inflamed via integrins and cytokines (seen with IVDU)

platelet and thrombin deposition

leads to fibrin formation

vegetation (aka coagulum) forms on the valve

vegetation becomes nidus for infection via bacteremia (usually transient)

bacteria enter circulation via:
• mucosal membranes
• skin
• focal infections

bacterial infection activates inflammatory response

Staphylococcus aureus (most common)
Streptococcus sanguis, bovis, mutans, mitis
Enterococcus
HACEK organisms (Haemophilus, Actinobacillus, Cardiobacterium, Eikenella, Kingella)

these organisms are responsible for > 80% of infective endocarditis

vegetation increases in size as platelets and fibrin are deposited

bacteria are protected and able to proliferate within growing vegetation

nonspecific signs and symptoms:
• fever (most common)
• chills
• malaise
• nausea
• night sweats
• arthralgias
• myalgias
• weight loss

vegetation can embolize to different location

infection leads to clinical manifestations of **infective endocarditis**

activates both humoral and cellular immune responses (see maps)

bacteria resist host immune defenses and are able to disseminate

immune complex deposition can lead to

• glomerulonephritis
• immune complex vasculitis

4 broad classifications of endocarditis:
• native valve infections
• prosthetic valve infections
• infection from IVDU
• nosocomial infections

damage cardiac structures:
• valve destruction
• new or changing murmur
• heart failure
• pericarditis
• prosthetic valve endocarditis

complications of infective endocarditis

cutaneous findings

• Janeway lesions
• Roth spots
• Osler's nodes

persistent bacteremia

• septic joints
• sepsis (see map)

septic emboli

right sided infective endocarditis leads to pulmonary emboli (more common with IVDU)

left sided infective endocarditis leads to emboli of brain, spleen, kidney, gastrointestinal tract, extremities

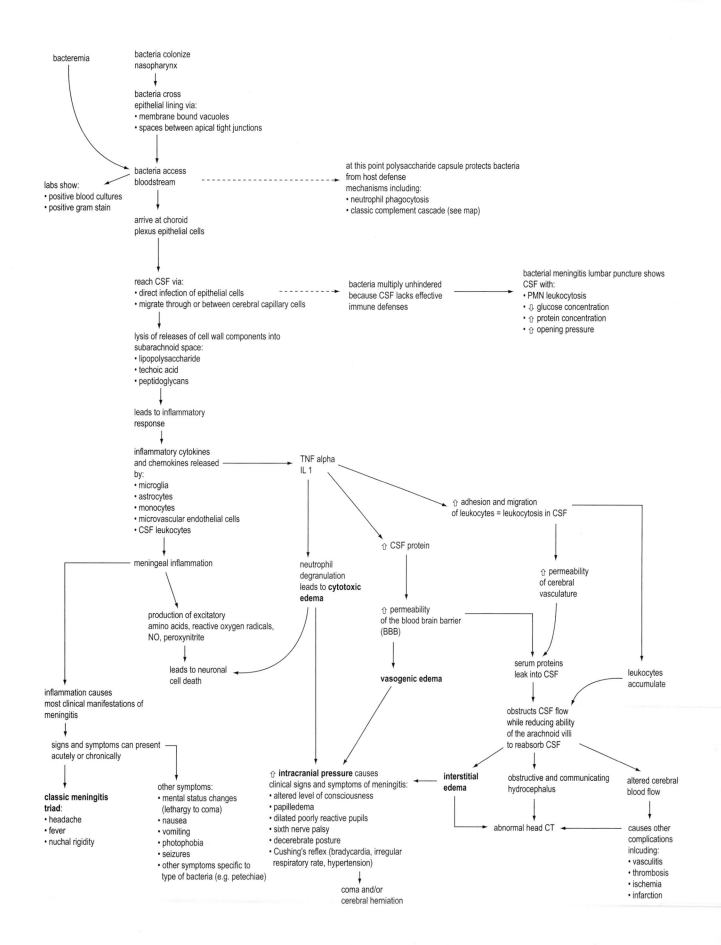

bacteremia

bacteria colonize
nasopharynx

bacteria cross
epithelial lining via:
• membrane bound vacuoles
• spaces between apical tight junctions

bacteria access
bloodstream

at this point polysaccharide capsule protects bacteria
from host defense
mechanisms including:
• neutrophil phagocytosis
• classic complement cascade (see map)

labs show:
• positive blood cultures
• positive gram stain

arrive at choroid
plexus epithelial cells

reach CSF via:
• direct infection of epithelial cells
• migrate through or between cerebral capillary cells

bacteria multiply unhindered
because CSF lacks effective
immune defenses

bacterial meningitis lumbar puncture shows
CSF with:
• PMN leukocytosis
• ⇩ glucose concentration
• ⇧ protein concentration
• ⇧ opening pressure

lysis of releases of cell wall components into
subarachnoid space:
• lipopolysaccharide
• techoic acid
• peptidoglycans

leads to inflammatory
response

inflammatory cytokines
and chemokines released
by:
• microglia
• astrocytes
• monocytes
• microvascular endothelial cells
• CSF leukocytes

TNF alpha
IL 1

⇧ adhesion and migration
of leukocytes = leukocytosis in CSF

⇧ CSF protein

⇧ permeability
of cerebral
vasculature

meningeal inflammation

neutrophil
degranulation
leads to **cytotoxic
edema**

production of excitatory
amino acids, reactive oxygen radicals,
NO, peroxynitrite

⇧ permeability
of the blood brain barrier
(BBB)

serum proteins
leak into CSF

leukocytes
accumulate

leads to neuronal
cell death

vasogenic edema

inflammation causes
most clinical manifestations of
meningitis

obstructs CSF flow
while reducing ability
of the arachnoid villi
to reabsorb CSF

signs and symptoms can present
acutely or chronically

⇧ **intracranial pressure** causes
clinical signs and symptoms of meningitis:
• altered level of consciousness
• papilledema
• dilated poorly reactive pupils
• sixth nerve palsy
• decerebrate posture
• Cushing's reflex (bradycardia, irregular
  respiratory rate, hypertension)

**interstitial
edema**

obstructive and communicating
hydrocephalus

altered cerebral
blood flow

**classic meningitis
triad:**
• headache
• fever
• nuchal rigidity

other symptoms:
• mental status changes
  (lethargy to coma)
• nausea
• vomiting
• photophobia
• seizures
• other symptoms specific to
  type of bacteria (e.g. petechiae)

abnormal head CT

causes other
complications
inlcuding:
• vasculitis
• thrombosis
• ischemia
• infarction

coma and/or
cerebral herniation

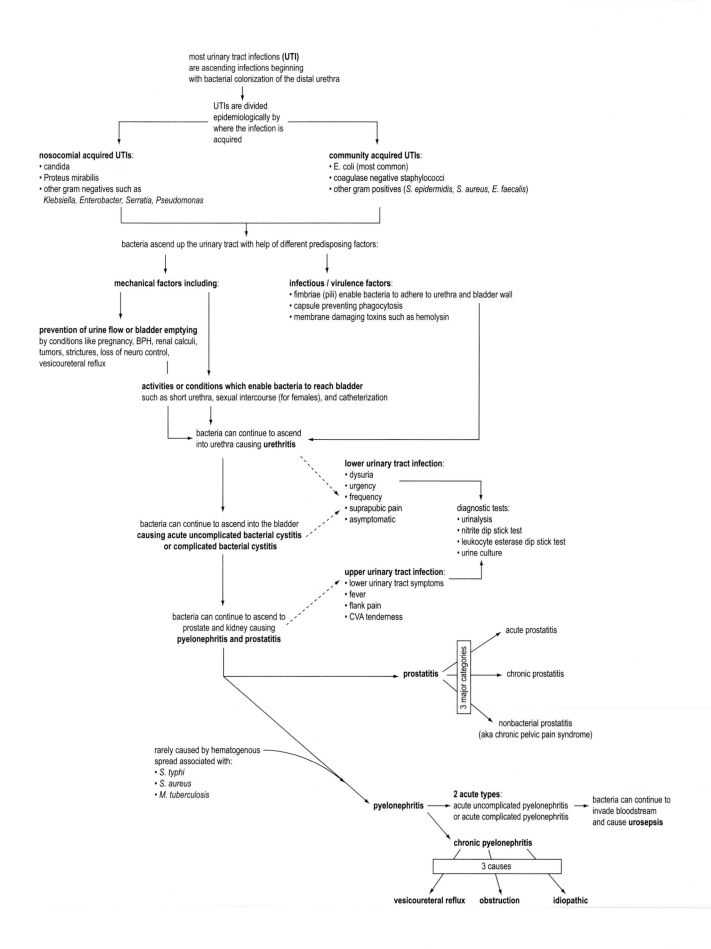

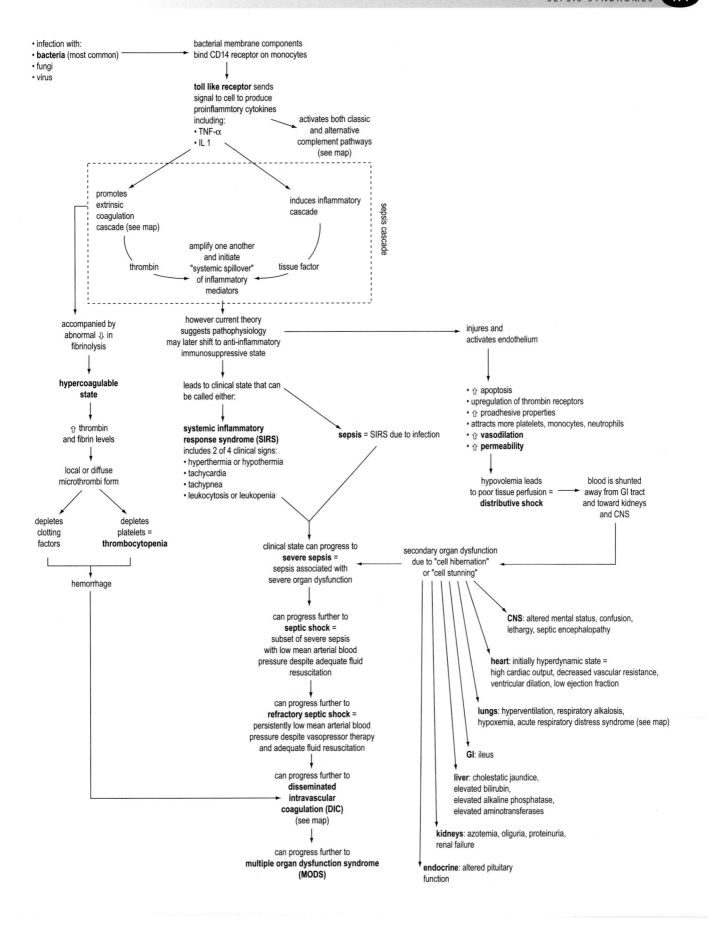

• infection with:
• **bacteria** (most common)
• fungi
• virus

bacterial membrane components bind CD14 receptor on monocytes

toll like receptor sends signal to cell to produce proinflammtory cytokines including:
• TNF-α
• IL 1

activates both classic and alternative complement pathways (see map)

promotes extrinsic coagulation cascade (see map)

induces inflammatory cascade

sepsis cascade

amplify one another and initiate "systemic spillover" of inflammatory mediators

thrombin

tissue factor

accompanied by abnormal ⇩ in fibrinolysis

however current theory suggests pathophysiology may later shift to anti-inflammatory immunosuppressive state

injures and activates endothelium

hypercoagulable state

⇧ thrombin and fibrin levels

local or diffuse microthrombi form

leads to clinical state that can be called either:

systemic inflammatory response syndrome (SIRS) includes 2 of 4 clinical signs:
• hyperthermia or hypothermia
• tachycardia
• tachypnea
• leukocytosis or leukopenia

sepsis = SIRS due to infection

• ⇧ apoptosis
• upregulation of thrombin receptors
• ⇧ proadhesive properties
• attracts more platelets, monocytes, neutrophils
• ⇧ **vasodilation**
• ⇧ **permeability**

hypovolemia leads to poor tissue perfusion = **distributive shock**

blood is shunted away from GI tract and toward kidneys and CNS

depletes clotting factors

depletes platelets = **thrombocytopenia**

hemorrhage

clinical state can progress to **severe sepsis** = sepsis associated with severe organ dysfunction

secondary organ dysfunction due to "cell hibernation" or "cell stunning"

CNS: altered mental status, confusion, lethargy, septic encephalopathy

can progress further to **septic shock** = subset of severe sepsis with low mean arterial blood pressure despite adequate fluid resuscitation

heart: initially hyperdynamic state = high cardiac output, decreased vascular resistance, ventricular dilation, low ejection fraction

can progress further to **refractory septic shock** = persistently low mean arterial blood pressure despite vasopressor therapy and adequate fluid resuscitation

lungs: hyperventilation, respiratory alkalosis, hypoxemia, acute respiratory distress syndrome (see map)

GI: ileus

can progress further to **disseminated intravascular coagulation (DIC)** (see map)

liver: cholestatic jaundice, elevated bilirubin, elevated alkaline phosphatase, elevated aminotransferases

kidneys: azotemia, oliguria, proteinuria, renal failure

can progress further to **multiple organ dysfunction syndrome (MODS)**

endocrine: altered pituitary function

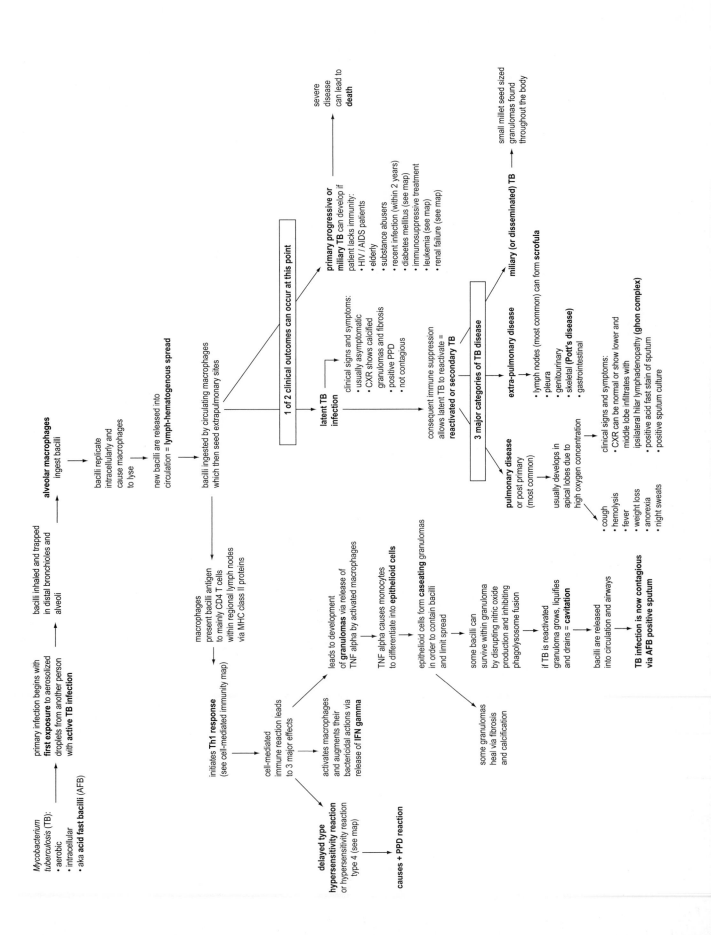

Mycobacterium tuberculosis (TB):
• aerobic
• intracellular
• aka **acid fast bacilli** (AFB)

primary infection begins with **first exposure** to aerosolized droplets from another person with **active TB infection**

bacilli inhaled and trapped in distal bronchioles and alveoli

alveolar macrophages ingest bacilli

bacilli replicate intracellularly and cause macrophages to lyse

new bacilli are released into circulation = **lymph-hematogenous spread**

bacilli ingested by circulating macrophages which then seed extrapulmonary sites

1 of 2 clinical outcomes can occur at this point

primary progressive or miliary TB can develop if patient lacks immunity:
• HIV / AIDS patients
• elderly
• substance abusers
• recent infection (within 2 years)
• diabetes mellitus (see map)
• immunosuppressive treatment
• leukemia (see map)
• renal failure (see map)

severe disease can lead to **death**

latent TB infection

clinical signs and symptoms:
• usually asymptomatic
• CXR shows calcified granulomas and fibrosis
• positive PPD
• not contagious

consequent immune suppression allows latent TB to reactivate = **reactivated or secondary TB**

3 major categories of TB disease

extra-pulmonary disease
• lymph nodes (most common) can form **scrofula**
• pleura
• genitourinary
• skeletal (**Pott's disease**)
• gastrointestinal

miliary (or disseminated) TB

small millet seed sized granulomas found throughout the body

pulmonary disease or post primary (most common)

usually develops in apical lobes due to high oxygen concentration

clinical signs and symptoms:
• CXR can be normal or show lower and middle lobe infiltrates with ipsilateral hilar lymphadenopathy (**ghon complex**)
• positive acid fast stain of sputum
• positive sputum culture

• cough
• hemolysis
• fever
• weight loss
• anorexia
• night sweats

macrophages present bacilli antigen to mainly CD4 T cells within regional lymph nodes via MHC class II proteins

initiates **Th1 response** (see cell-mediated immunity map)

cell-mediated immune reaction leads to 3 major effects

leads to development of **granulomas** via release of TNF alpha by activated macrophages

TNF alpha causes monocytes to differentiate into **epithelioid cells**

epithelioid cells form **caseating** granulomas in order to contain bacilli and limit spread

activates macrophages and augments their bactericidal actions via release of **IFN gamma**

some bacilli can survive within granuloma by disrupting nitric oxide production and inhibiting phagolysosome fusion

if TB is reactivated granuloma grows, liquifies and drains = **cavitation**

bacilli are released into circulation and airways

TB infection is now contagious via AFB positive sputum

delayed type hypersensitivity reaction or hypersensitivity reaction type 4 (see map)

causes + PPD reaction

some granulomas heal via fibrosis and calcification

Endocrine Disorders

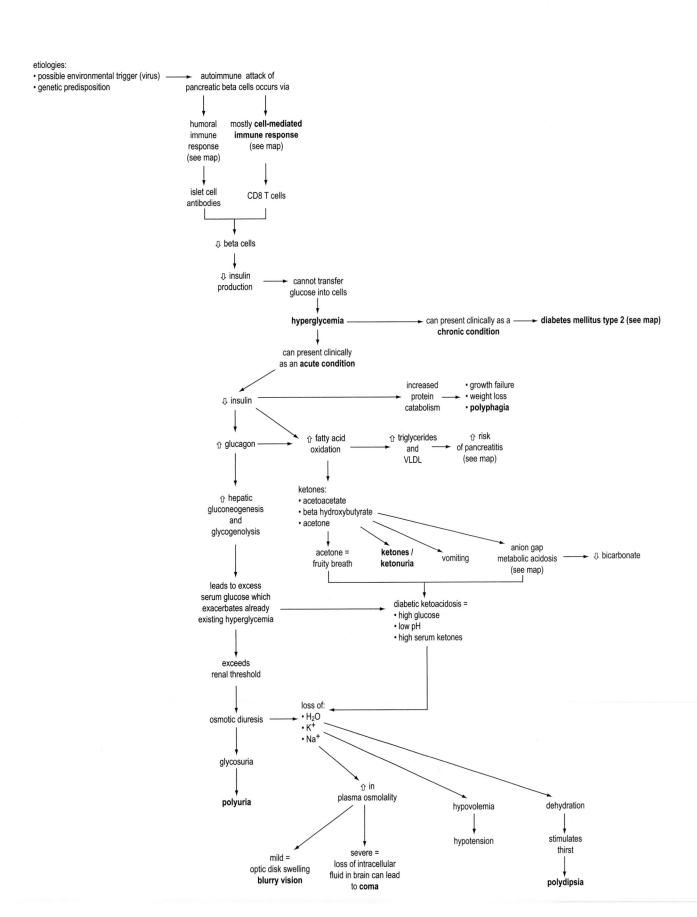

etiologies:
• possible environmental trigger (virus) ⟶ autoimmune attack of
• genetic predisposition   pancreatic beta cells occurs via

humoral   mostly **cell-mediated**
immune   **immune response**
response   (see map)
(see map)

islet cell   CD8 T cells
antibodies

⇩ beta cells

⇩ insulin ⟶ cannot transfer
production   glucose into cells

hyperglycemia ⟶ can present clinically as a ⟶ **diabetes mellitus type 2 (see map)**
                        chronic condition

can present clinically
as an **acute condition**

⇩ insulin ⟶ increased ⟶ • growth failure
              protein   • weight loss
              catabolism   • **polyphagia**

⇧ glucagon ⟶ ⇧ fatty acid ⟶ ⇧ triglycerides ⟶ ⇧ risk
              oxidation   and   of pancreatitis
                              VLDL   (see map)

⇧ hepatic   ketones:
gluconeogenesis   • acetoacetate
and   • beta hydroxybutyrate
glycogenolysis   • acetone

                       acetone =   **ketones /**   vomiting   anion gap ⟶ ⇩ bicarbonate
                       fruity breath   **ketonuria**   metabolic acidosis
                                                                       (see map)

leads to excess
serum glucose which ⟶   diabetic ketoacidosis =
exacerbates already   • high glucose
existing hyperglycemia   • low pH
                                        • high serum ketones

exceeds
renal threshold

                       loss of:
                       • H$_2$O
osmotic diuresis ⟶   • K$^+$
                       • Na$^+$

glycosuria

                       ⇧ in   hypovolemia   dehydration
polyuria   plasma osmolality
                                                     hypotension   stimulates
                                                                    thirst

            mild =   severe =
            optic disk swelling loss of intracellular   **polydipsia**
            blurry vision   fluid in brain can lead
                                 to **coma**

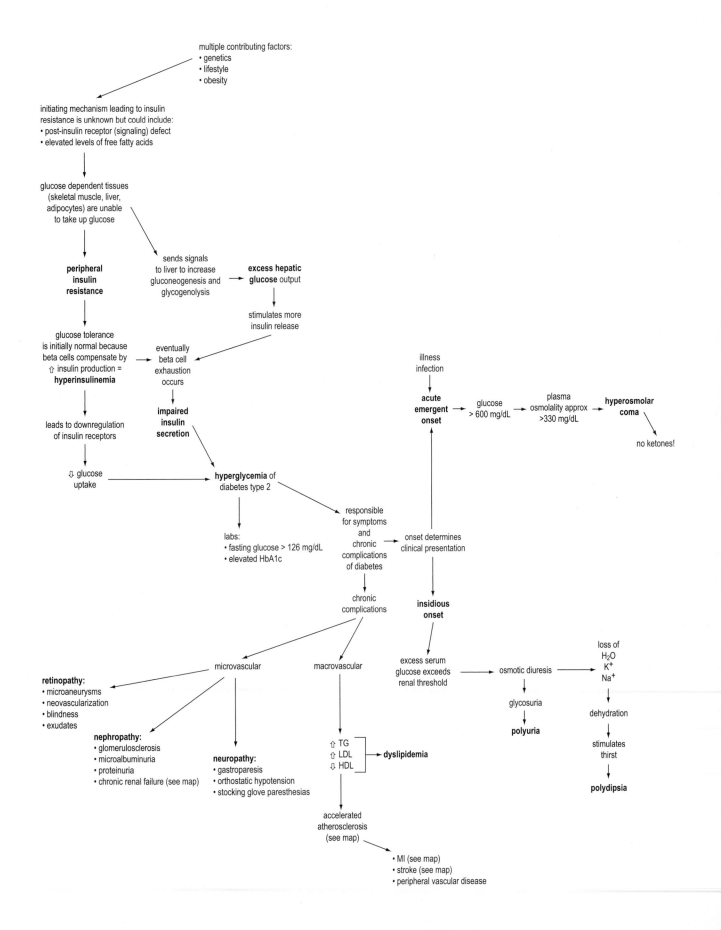

multiple contributing factors:
• genetics
• lifestyle
• obesity

initiating mechanism leading to insulin
resistance is unknown but could include:
• post-insulin receptor (signaling) defect
• elevated levels of free fatty acids

glucose dependent tissues
(skeletal muscle, liver,
adipocytes) are unable
to take up glucose

**peripheral
insulin
resistance**

sends signals
to liver to increase
gluconeogenesis and
glycogenolysis

**excess hepatic
glucose** output

stimulates more
insulin release

glucose tolerance
is initially normal because
beta cells compensate by
⇧ insulin production =
hyperinsulinemia

eventually
beta cell
exhaustion
occurs

illness
infection

**acute
emergent
onset**

glucose
> 600 mg/dL

plasma
osmolality approx
>330 mg/dL

**hyperosmolar
coma**

no ketones!

leads to downregulation
of insulin receptors

**impaired
insulin
secretion**

⇩ glucose
uptake

hyperglycemia of
diabetes type 2

labs:
• fasting glucose > 126 mg/dL
• elevated HbA1c

responsible
for symptoms
and
chronic
complications
of diabetes

onset determines
clinical presentation

chronic
complications

**insidious
onset**

microvascular

macrovascular

excess serum
glucose exceeds
renal threshold

osmotic diuresis

loss of
H$_2$O
K$^+$
Na$^+$

retinopathy:
• microaneurysms
• neovascularization
• blindness
• exudates

glycosuria

polyuria

dehydration

nephropathy:
• glomerulosclerosis
• microalbuminuria
• proteinuria
• chronic renal failure (see map)

neuropathy:
• gastroparesis
• orthostatic hypotension
• stocking glove paresthesias

⇧ TG
⇧ LDL
⇩ HDL

dyslipidemia

stimulates
thirst

polydipsia

accelerated
atherosclerosis
(see map)

• MI (see map)
• stroke (see map)
• peripheral vascular disease

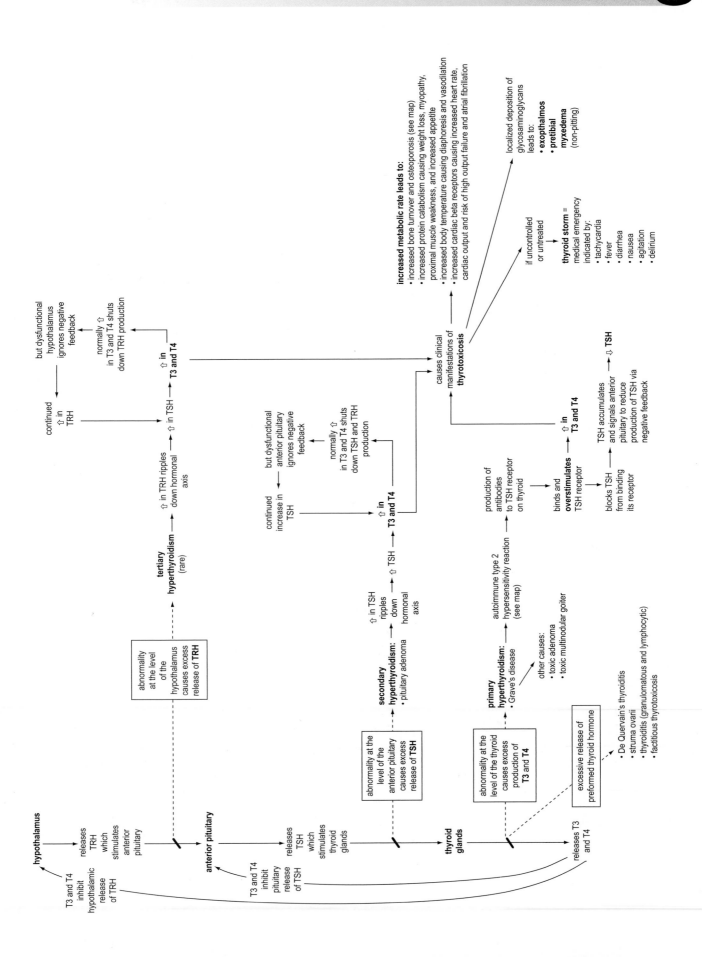

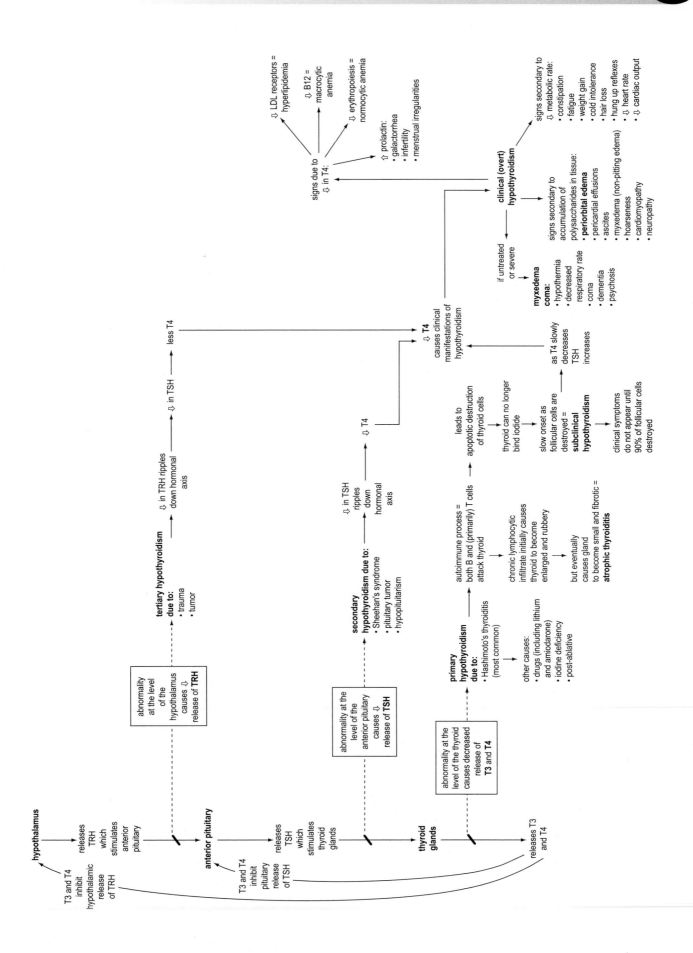

hypothalamus

T3 and T4 inhibit hypothalamic release of TRH

releases TRH which stimulates anterior pituitary

abnormality at the level of the hypothalamus causes ⇩ release of **TRH**

tertiary hypothyroidism
due to:
• trauma
• tumor

⇩ in TRH ripples down hormonal axis ⟶ ⇩ in TSH ⟶ less T4

anterior pituitary

T3 and T4 inhibit pituitary release of TSH

releases TSH which stimulates thyroid glands

abnormality at the level of the anterior pituitary causes ⇩ release of **TSH**

secondary
hypothyroidism due to:
• Sheehan's syndrome
• pituitary tumor
• hypopituitarism

⇩ in TSH ripples down hormonal axis ⟶ ⇩ T4

thyroid glands

releases T3 and T4

abnormality at the level of the thyroid causes decreased release of **T3 and T4**

primary
hypothyroidism
due to:
• Hashimoto's thyroiditis (most common)

other causes:
• drugs (including lithium and amiodarone)
• iodine deficiency
• post-ablative

autoimmune process = both B and (primarily) T cells attack thyroid

chronic lymphocytic infiltrate initially causes thyroid to become enlarged and rubbery

but eventually causes gland to become small and fibrotic = **atrophic thyroiditis**

leads to apoptotic destruction of thyroid cells

thyroid can no longer bind iodide

slow onset as follicular cells are destroyed = **subclinical hypothyroidism**

clinical symptoms do not appear until 90% of follicular cells destroyed

as T4 slowly decreases TSH increases

⇩ **T4** causes clinical manifestations of hypothyroidism

signs due to ⇩ in T4:

⇩ LDL receptors = hyperlipidemia

⇩ B12 = macrocytic anemia

⇩ erythropoiesis = normocytic anemia

⇧ prolactin:
• galactorrhea
• infertility
• menstrual irregularities

clinical (overt)
hypothyroidism

signs secondary to ⇩ metabolic rate:
• constipation
• fatigue
• weight gain
• cold intolerance
• hair loss
• hung up reflexes
• ⇩ heart rate
• ⇩ cardiac output

signs secondary to accumulation of polysaccharides in tissue:
• **periorbital edema**
• pericardial effusions
• ascites
• myxedema (non-pitting edema)
• hoarseness
• cardiomyopathy
• neuropathy

if untreated or severe

myxedema coma:
• hypothermia
• decreased respiratory rate
• coma
• dementia
• psychosis

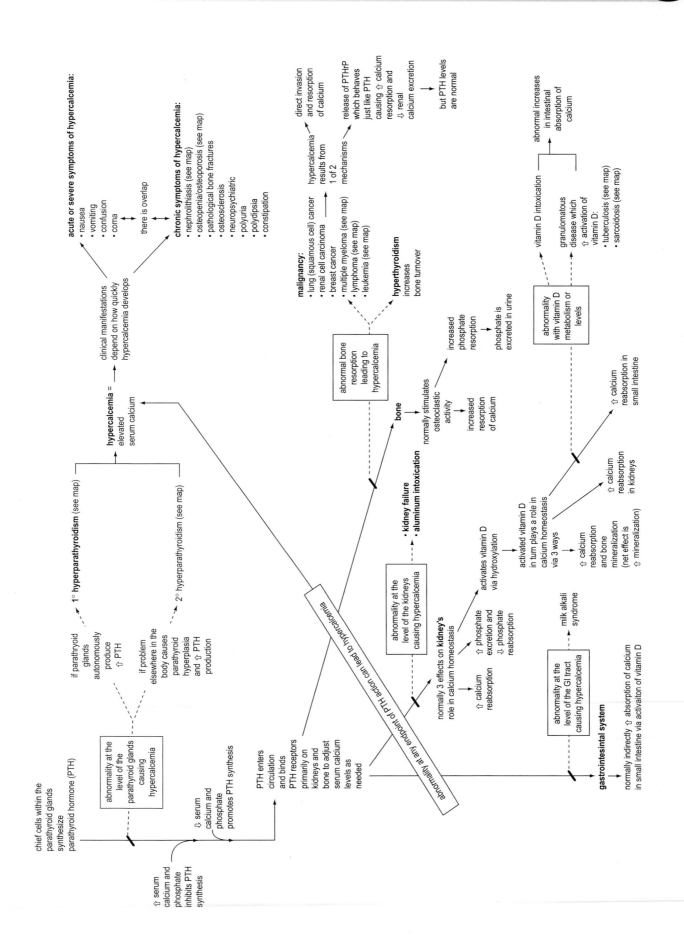

acute or severe symptoms of hypercalcemia:
- nausea
- vomiting
- confusion
- coma

there is overlap ←→

chronic symptoms of hypercalcemia:
- nephrolithiasis (see map)
- osteopenia/osteoporosis (see map)
- pathological bone fractures
- osteosclerosis
- neuropsychiatric
- polyuria
- polydipsia
- constipation

clinical manifestations depend on how quickly hypercalcemia develops

hypercalcemia = elevated serum calcium

direct invasion and resorption of calcium

release of PTHrP which behaves just like PTH causing ⇧ calcium resorption and ⇩ renal calcium excretion → but PTH levels are normal

hypercalcemia results from 1 of 2 mechanisms

malignancy:
- lung (squamous cell cancer)
- renal cell carcinoma
- breast cancer
- multiple myeloma (see map)
- lymphoma (see map)
- leukemia (see map)

hyperthyroidism increases bone turnover

abnormal bone resorption leading to hypercalcemia

bone normally stimulates osteoclastic activity

increased phosphate resorption

increased resorption of calcium

phosphate is excreted in urine

abnormal increases in intestinal absorption of calcium

vitamin D intoxication

granulomatous disease which ⇧ activation of vitamin D:
- tuberculosis (see map)
- sarcoidosis (see map)

abnormality with vitamin D metabolism or levels

1° **hyperparathyroidism** (see map)

2° hyperparathyroidism (see map)

• kidney failure • aluminum intoxication

activates vitamin D via hydroxylation

activated vitamin D in turn plays a role in calcium homeostasis via 3 ways

⇧ calcium reabsorption and bone mineralization (net effect is ⇧ mineralization)

⇧ calcium reabsorption in kidneys

⇧ calcium reabsorption in small intestine

abnormality at the level of the kidneys causing hypercalcemia

kidney's

normally 3 effects on calcium homeostasis

⇧ calcium reabsorption

⇧ phosphate excretion and ⇩ phosphate reabsorption

milk alkali syndrome

abnormality at the level of the GI tract causing hypercalcemia

abnormality at any endpoint of PTH action can lead to hypercalcemia

abnormality at the level of the parathyroid glands causing hypercalcemia

if parathyroid glands autonomously produce ⇧ PTH

if problem elsewhere in the body causes parathyroid hyperplasia and ⇧ PTH production

chief cells within the parathyroid glands synthesize parathyroid hormone (PTH)

⇧ serum calcium and phosphate inhibits PTH synthesis

⇩ serum calcium and phosphate promotes PTH synthesis

PTH enters circulation and binds PTH receptors primarily on kidneys and bone to adjust serum calcium levels as needed

gastrointestinal system

normally indirectly ⇧ absorption of calcium in small intestine via activation of vitamin D

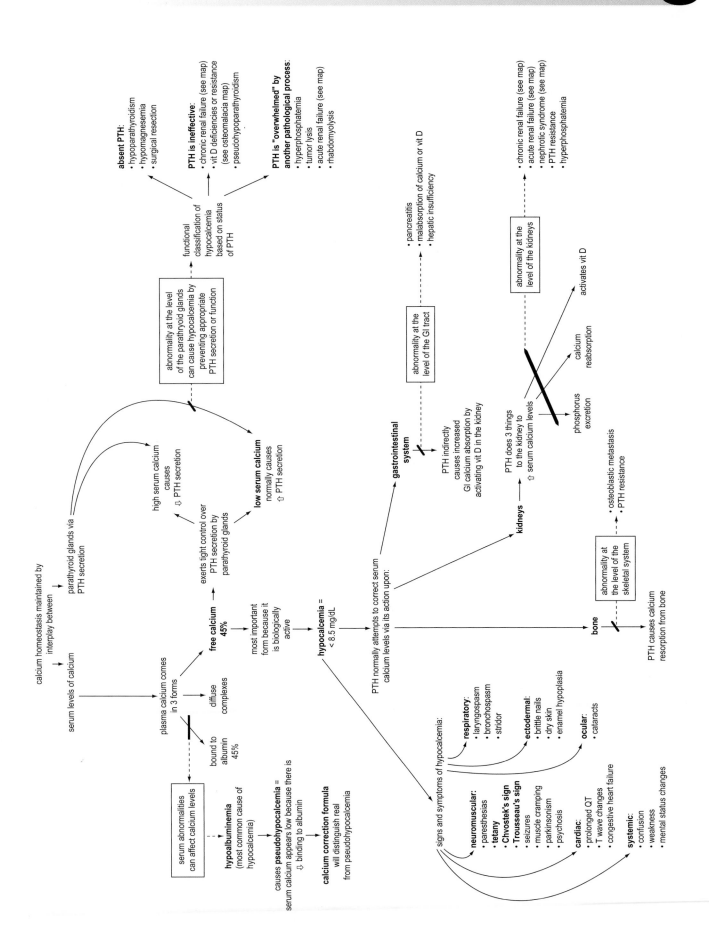

calcium homeostasis maintained by interplay between

parathyroid glands via PTH secretion

serum levels of calcium

plasma calcium comes in 3 forms

free calcium 45%

diffuse complexes

bound to albumin 45%

high serum calcium causes ⇩ PTH secretion

exerts tight control over PTH secretion by parathyroid glands

low serum calcium normally causes ⇧ PTH secretion

most important form because it is biologically active

serum abnormalities can affect calcium levels

hypoalbuminemia (most common cause of hypocalcemia)

causes **pseudohypocalcemia** = serum calcium appears low because there is ⇩ binding to albumin

calcium correction formula will distinguish real from pseudohypocalcemia

hypocalcemia = < 8.5 mg/dL

abnormality at the level of the parathyroid glands can cause hypocalcemia by preventing appropriate PTH secretion or function

functional classification of hypocalcemia based on status of PTH

absent PTH:
• hypoparathyroidism
• hypomagnesemia
• surgical resection

PTH is ineffective:
• chronic renal failure (see map)
• vit D deficiencies or resistance (see osteomalacia map)
• pseudohypoparathyroidism

PTH is "overwhelmed" by another pathological process:
• hyperphosphatemia
• tumor lysis
• acute renal failure (see map)
• rhabdomyolysis

PTH normally attempts to correct serum calcium levels via its action upon:

gastrointestinal system

kidneys

bone

abnormality at the level of the GI tract

• pancreatitis
• malabsorption of calcium or vit D
• hepatic insufficiency

PTH indirectly causes increased GI calcium absorption by activating vit D in the kidney

PTH does 3 things to the kidney to ⇧ serum calcium levels

abnormality at the level of the kidneys

• chronic renal failure (see map)
• acute renal failure (see map)
• nephrotic syndrome (see map)
• PTH resistance
• hyperphosphatemia

phosphorus excretion

calcium reabsorption

activates vit D

abnormality at the level of the skeletal system

• osteoblastic metastasis
• PTH resistance

PTH causes calcium resorption from bone

signs and symptoms of hypocalcemia:

respiratory:
• laryngospasm
• bronchospasm
• stridor

ectodermal:
• brittle nails
• dry skin
• enamel hypoplasia

ocular:
• cataracts

neuromuscular:
• paresthesias
• **tetany**
• **Chvostek's sign**
• **Trousseau's sign**
• seizures
• muscle cramping
• parkinsonism
• psychosis

cardiac:
• prolonged QT
• T wave changes
• congestive heart failure

systemic:
• confusion
• weakness
• mental status changes

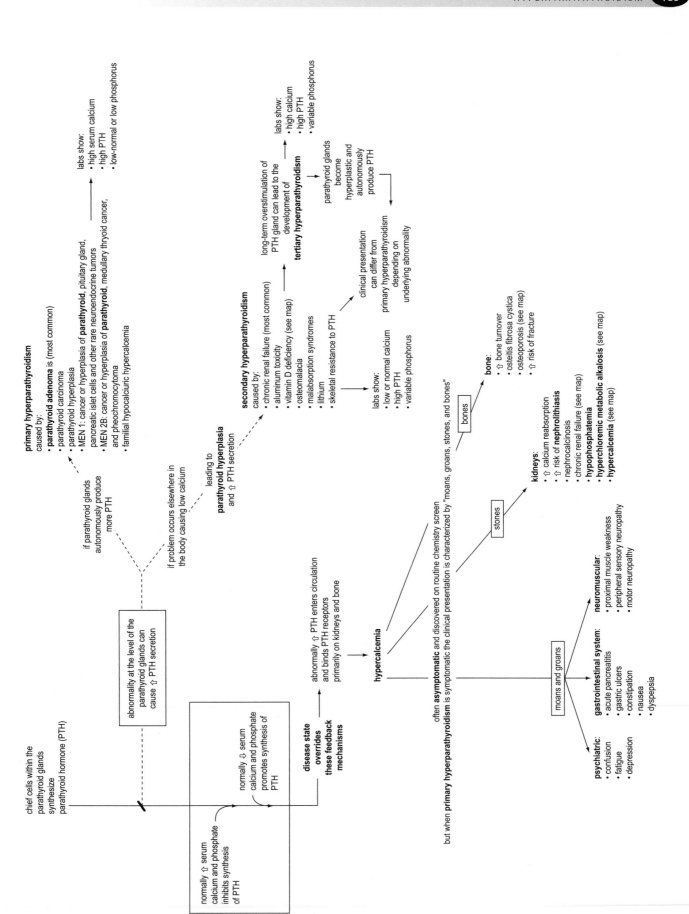

chief cells within the parathyroid glands synthesize parathyroid hormone (PTH)

normally ⇧ serum calcium and phosphate inhibits synthesis of PTH

normally ⇩ serum calcium and phosphate promotes synthesis of PTH

disease state overrides these feedback mechanisms

abnormality at the level of the parathyroid glands can cause ⇧ PTH secretion

if parathyroid glands autonomously produce more PTH

if problem occurs elsewhere in the body causing low calcium

leading to

parathyroid hyperplasia and ⇧ PTH secretion

primary hyperparathyroidism
caused by:
• **parathyroid adenoma** is (most common)
• parathyroid carcinoma
• parathyroid hyperplasia
• MEN 1: cancer or hyperplasia of **parathyroid**, pituitary gland, pancreatic islet cells and other rare neuroendocrine tumors
• MEN 2B: cancer or hyperplasia of **parathyroid**, medullary thryoid cancer, and pheochromocytoma
• familial hypocalciuric hypercalcemia

labs show:
• high serum calcium
• high PTH
• low-normal or low phosphorus

secondary hyperparathyroidism
caused by:
• chronic renal failure (most common)
• aluminum toxicity
• vitamin D deficiency (see map)
• osteomalacia
• malabsorption syndromes
• lithium
• skeletal resistance to PTH

labs show:
• low or normal calcium
• high PTH
• variable phosphorus

long-term overstimulation of PTH gland can lead to the development of **tertiary hyperparathyroidism**

parathyroid glands become hyperplastic and autonomously produce PTH

labs show:
• high calcium
• high PTH
• variable phosphorus

clinical presentation can differ from primary hyperparathyroidism depending on underlying abnormality

abnormally ⇧ PTH enters circulation and binds PTH receptors primarily on kidneys and bone

hypercalcemia

often **asymptomatic** and discovered on routine chemistry screen
but when **primary hyperparathyroidism** is symptomatic the clinical presentation is characterized by "moans, groans, stones, and bones"

bones

stones

moans and groans

bone:
• ⇧ bone turnover
• osteitis fibrosa cystica
• osteoporosis (see map)
• ⇧ risk of fracture

kidneys:
• ⇧ calcium reabsorption
• ⇧ risk of **nephrolithiasis**
• nephrocalcinosis
• chronic renal failure (see map)
• **hypophosphatemia**
• **hyperchloremic metabolic alkalosis** (see map)
• **hypercalcemia** (see map)

neuromuscular:
• proximal muscle weakness
• peripheral sensory neuropathy
• motor neuropathy

gastrointestinal system:
• acute pancreatitis
• gastric ulcers
• constipation
• nausea
• dyspepsia

psychiatric:
• confusion
• fatigue
• depression

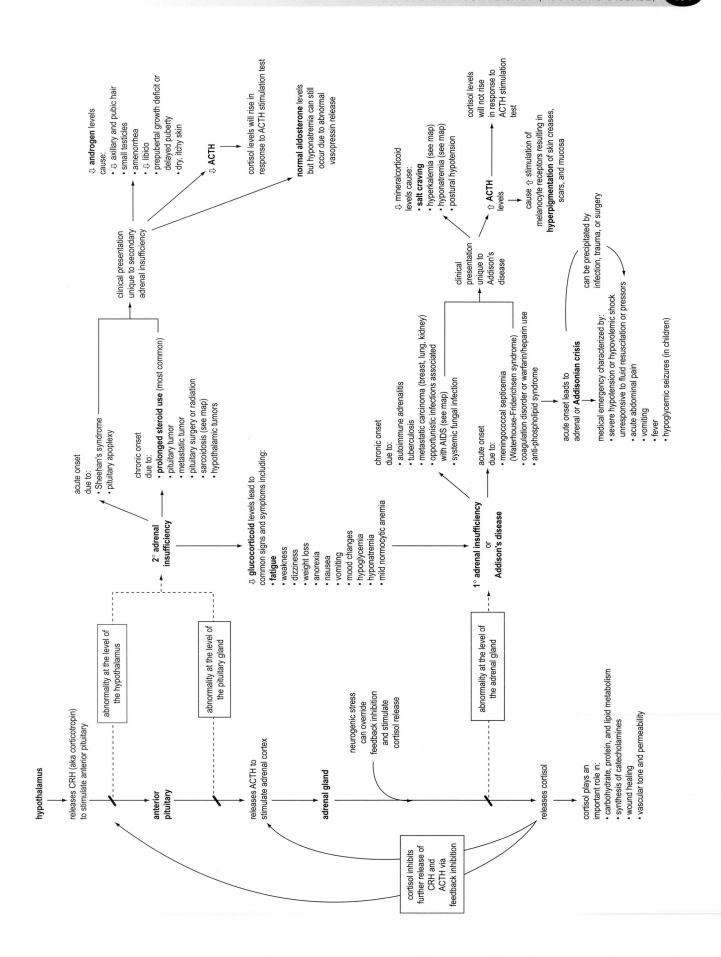

hypothalamus

releases CRH (aka corticotropin) to stimulate anterior pituitary

abnormality at the level of the hypothalamus

anterior pituitary

abnormality at the level of the pituitary gland

releases ACTH to stimulate adrenal cortex

adrenal gland

neurogenic stress can override feedback inhibition and stimulate cortisol release

abnormality at the level of the adrenal gland

releases cortisol

cortisol plays an important role in:
- carbohydrate, protein, and lipid metabolism
- synthesis of catecholamines
- wound healing
- vascular tone and permeability

cortisol inhibits further release of CRH and ACTH via feedback inhibition

2° adrenal insufficiency

acute onset due to:
- Sheehan's syndrome
- pituitary apoplexy

chronic onset due to:
- **prolonged steroid use** (most common)
- pituitary tumor
- metastatic tumor
- pituitary surgery or radiation
- sarcoidosis (see map)
- hypothalamic tumors

⇓ **glucocorticoid** levels lead to common signs and symptoms including:
- **fatigue**
- weakness
- dizziness
- weight loss
- anorexia
- nausea
- vomiting
- mood changes
- hypoglycemia
- hyponatremia
- mild normocytic anemia

clinical presentation unique to secondary adrenal insufficiency

⇓ **androgen** levels cause:
- ⇓ axillary and pubic hair
- small testicles
- ⇓ libido
- amenorrhea
- prepubertal growth deficit or delayed puberty
- dry, itchy skin

⇓ **ACTH**

cortisol levels will rise in response to ACTH stimulation test

normal aldosterone levels but hyponatremia can still occur due to abnormal vasopressin release

1° adrenal insufficiency or **Addison's disease**

chronic onset due to:
- autoimmune adrenalitis
- tuberculosis
- metastatic carcinoma (breast, lung, kidney)
- opportunistic infections associated with AIDS (see map)
- systemic fungal infection

acute onset due to:
- meningococcal septicemia (Waterhouse-Friderichsen syndrome)
- coagulation disorder or warfarin/heparin use
- anti-phospholipid syndrome

acute onset leads to adrenal or **Addisonian crisis**

medical emergency characterized by:
- severe hypotension or hypovolemic shock unresponsive to fluid resuscitation or pressors
- acute abdominal pain
- vomiting
- fever
- hypoglycemic seizures (in children)

can be precipitated by infection, trauma, or surgery

clinical presentation unique to Addison's disease

⇓ mineralocorticoid levels cause:
- **salt craving**
- hyperkalemia (see map)
- hyponatremia (see map)
- postural hypotension

⇑ **ACTH** levels

cause ⇑ stimulation of melanocyte receptors resulting in **hyperpigmentation** of skin creases, scars, and mucosa

cortisol levels will not rise in response to ACTH stimulation test

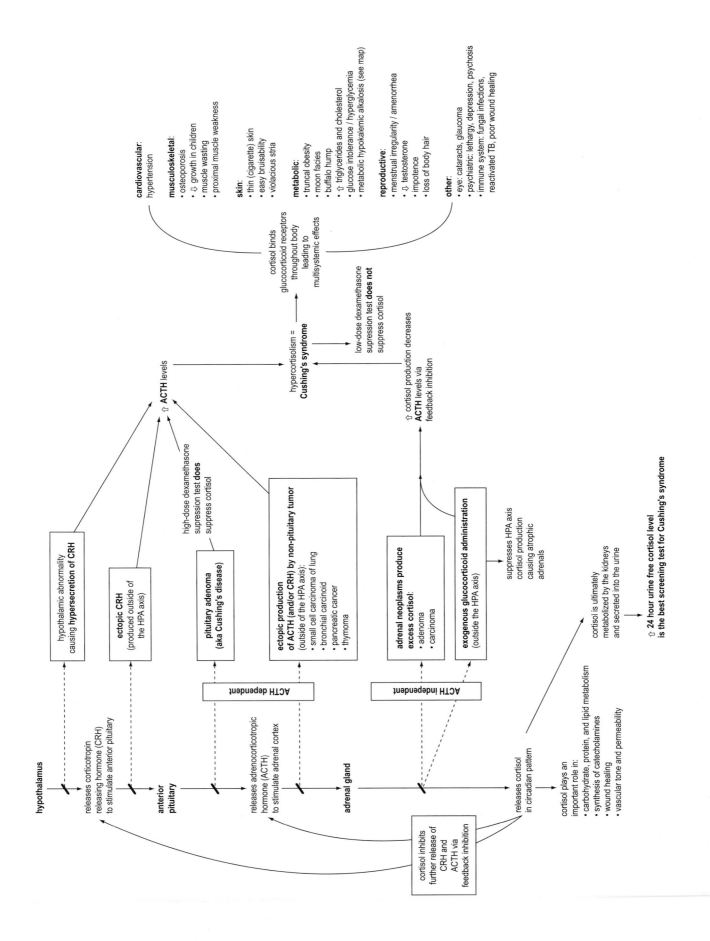

cardiovascular: hypertension

musculoskeletal:
• osteoporosis
• ⇩ growth in children
• muscle wasting
• proximal muscle weakness

skin:
• thin (cigarette) skin
• easy bruisability
• violacious stria

metabolic:
• truncal obesity
• moon facies
• buffalo hump
• ⇧ triglycerides and cholesterol
• glucose intolerance / hyperglycemia
• metabolic hypokalemic alkalosis (see map)

reproductive:
• menstrual irregularity / amenorrhea
• ⇩ testosterone
• impotence
• loss of body hair

other:
• eye: cataracts, glaucoma
• psychiatric: lethargy, depression, psychosis
• immune system: fungal infections, reactivated TB, poor wound healing

cortisol binds glucocorticoid receptors throughout body leading to multisystemic effects

hypercortisolism = **Cushing's syndrome**

low-dose dexamethasone supression test **does not** suppress cortisol

⇧ ACTH levels

⇧ cortisol production decreases **ACTH** levels via feedback inhibition

high-dose dexamethasone supression test **does** suppress cortisol

hypothalamic abnormality causing **hypersecretion of CRH**

ectopic CRH (produced outside of the HPA axis)

pituitary adenoma (aka Cushing's disease)

ectopic production of ACTH (and/or CRH) by non-pituitary tumor (outside of the HPA axis):
• small cell carcinoma of lung
• bronchial carcinoid
• pancreatic cancer
• thymoma

ACTH dependent

adrenal neoplasms produce excess cortisol:
• adenoma
• carcinoma

exogenous glucocorticoid administration (outside the HPA axis)

ACTH independent

suppresses HPA axis cortisol production causing atrophic adrenals

hypothalamus

releases corticotropin releasing hormone (CRH) to stimulate anterior pituitary

anterior pituitary

releases adrenocorticotropic hormone (ACTH) to stimulate adrenal cortex

adrenal gland

releases cortisol in circadian pattern

cortisol plays an important role in:
• carbohydrate, protein, and lipid metabolism
• synthesis of catecholamines
• wound healing
• vascular tone and permeability

cortisol inhibits further release of CRH and ACTH via feedback inhibition

cortisol is ultimately metabolized by the kidneys and secreted into the urine

⇧ **24 hour urine free cortisol level is the best screening test for Cushing's syndrome**

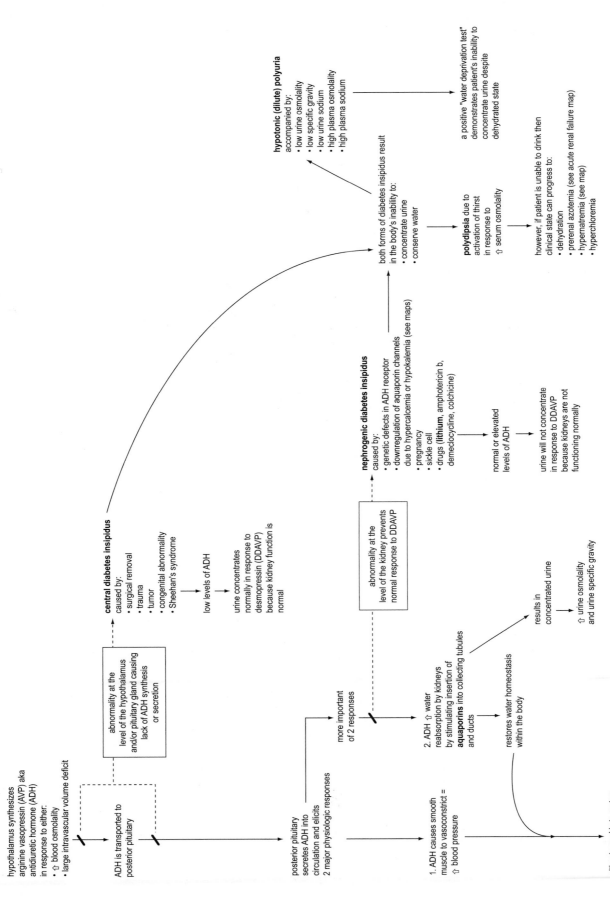

hypothalamus synthesizes arginine vasopressin (AVP) aka antidiuretic hormone (ADH) in response to either:
• ⇧ blood osmolality
• large intravascular volume deficit

ADH is transported to posterior pituitary

posterior pituitary secretes ADH into circulation and elicits 2 major physiologic responses

1. ADH causes smooth muscle to vasoconstrict = ⇧ blood pressure

more important of 2 responses

2. ADH ⇧ water reabsorption by kidneys by stimulating insertion of **aquaporins** into collecting tubules and ducts

restores water homeostasis within the body

ultimate goal is to restore perfusion when the body is confronted with volume deficits

abnormality at the level of the hypothalamus and/or pituitary gland causing lack of ADH synthesis or secretion

central diabetes insipidus
caused by:
• surgical removal
• trauma
• tumor
• congenital abnormality
• Sheehan's syndrome

low levels of ADH

urine concentrates normally in response to desmopressin (DDAVP) because kidney function is normal

abnormality at the level of the kidney prevents normal response to DDAVP

nephrogenic diabetes insipidus
caused by:
• genetic defects in ADH receptor
• downregulation of aquaporin channels due to hypercalcemia or hypokalemia (see maps)
• pregnancy
• sickle cell
• drugs (**lithium**, amphotericin b, demeclocycline, colchicine)

normal or elevated levels of ADH

urine will not concentrate in response to DDAVP because kidneys are not functioning normally

results in concentrated urine

⇧ urine osmolality and urine specific gravity

both forms of diabetes insipidus result in the body's inability to:
• concentrate urine
• conserve water

hypotonic (dilute) polyuria
accompanied by:
• low urine osmolality
• low specific gravity
• low urine sodium
• high plasma osmolality
• high plasma sodium

a positive "water deprivation test" demonstrates patient's inability to concentrate urine despite dehydrated state

polydipsia due to activation of thirst in response to ⇧ serum osmolality

however, if patient is unable to drink then clinical state can progress to:
• dehydration
• prerenal azotemia (see acute renal failure map)
• hypernatremia (see map)
• hyperchloremia

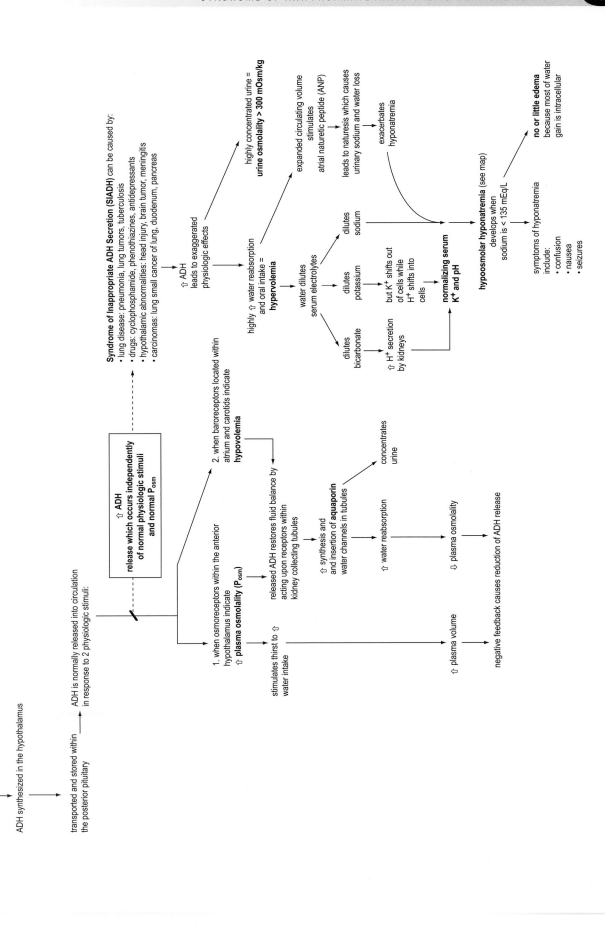

normal water homeostasis

closely associated with antidiuretic hormone (ADH) or arginine vasopressin (AVP)

ADH synthesized in the hypothalamus

transported and stored within the posterior pituitary

ADH is normally released into circulation in response to 2 physiologic stimuli:

⇧ ADH release which occurs independently of normal physiologic stimuli and normal P$_{osm}$

1. when osmoreceptors within the anterior hypothalamus indicate ⇧ **plasma osmolality (P$_{osm}$)**

2. when baroreceptors located within atrium and carotids indicate **hypovolemia**

stimulates thirst to ⇧ water intake

released ADH restores fluid balance by acting upon receptors within kidney collecting tubules

⇧ synthesis and and insertion of **aquaporin** water channels in tubules

concentrates urine

⇧ water reabsorption

⇩ plasma osmolality

⇧ plasma volume

negative feedback causes reduction of ADH release

Syndrome of Inappropriate ADH Secretion (SIADH) can be caused by:
- lung disease: pneumonia, lung tumors, tuberculosis
- drugs: cyclophosphamide, phenothiazines, antidepressants
- hypothalamic abnormalities: head injury, brain tumor, meningitis
- carcinomas: lung small cancer of lung, duodenum, pancreas

⇧ ADH leads to exaggerated physiologic effects

highly concentrated urine = **urine osmolality > 300 mOsm/kg**

highly ⇧ water reabsorption and oral intake = **hypervolemia**

expanded circulating volume stimulates atrial naturetic peptide (ANP)

leads to naturesis which causes urinary sodium and water loss

exacerbates hyponatremia

water dilutes serum electrolytes

dilutes sodium

dilutes potassium

but K$^+$ shifts out of cells while H$^+$ shifts into cells

dilutes bicarbonate

⇧ H$^+$ secretion by kidneys

normalizing serum K$^+$ and pH

hypoosmolar hyponatremia (see map) develops when sodium is < 135 mEq/L

symptoms of hyponatremia include:
- confusion
- nausea
- seizures

no or little edema because most of water gain is intracellular

Rheumatologic and Bone Disorders

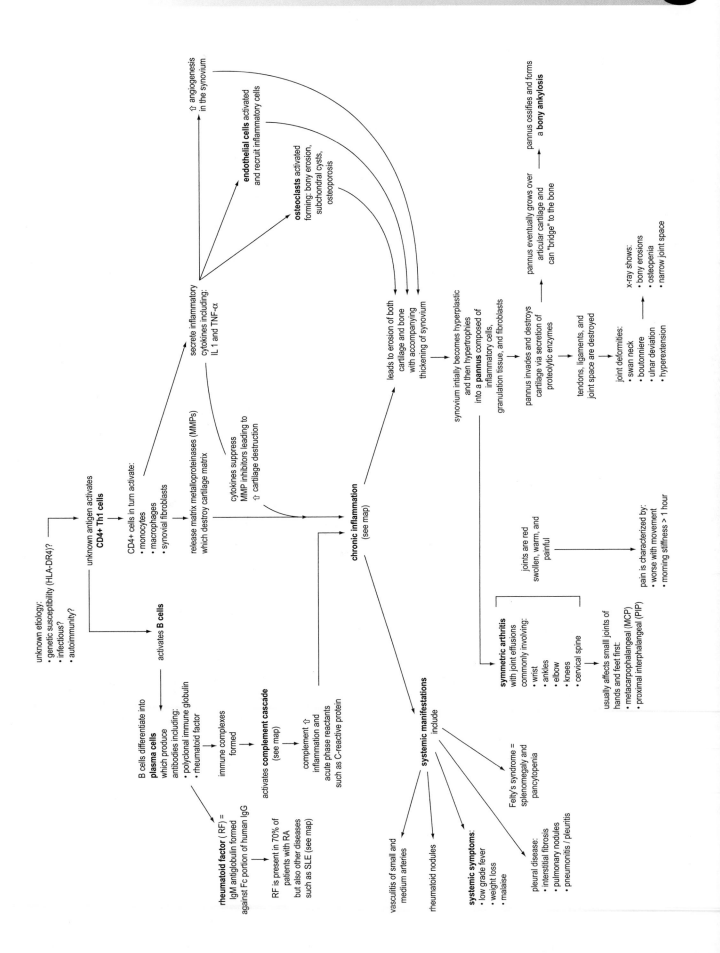

unknown etiology:
• genetic susceptibility (HLA-DR4)?
• infectious?
• autoimmunity?

unknown antigen activates
CD4+ Th1 cells

CD4+ cells in turn activate:
• monocytes
• macrophages
• synovial fibroblasts

secrete inflammatory
cytokines including:
IL 1 and TNF-α

↑ angiogenesis
in the synovium

endothelial cells activated
and recruit inflammatory cells

osteoclasts activated
forming: bony erosion,
subchondral cysts,
osteoporosis

release matrix metalloproteinases (MMPs)
which destroy cartilage matrix

cytokines suppress
MMP inhibitors leading to
↑ cartilage destruction

leads to erosion of both
cartilage and bone
with accompanying
thickening of synovium

synovium initially becomes hyperplastic
and then hypertrophies
into a **pannus** composed of
inflammatory cells,
granulation tissue, and fibroblasts

pannus invades and destroys
cartilage via secretion of
proteolytic enzymes

pannus eventually grows over
articular cartilage and
can "bridge" to the bone

pannus ossifies and forms → a **bony ankylosis**

tendons, ligaments, and
joint space are destroyed

joint deformities:
• swan neck
• boutonniere
• ulnar deviation
• hyperextension

x-ray shows:
• bony erosions
• osteopenia
• narrow joint space

activates **B cells**

B cells differentiate into
plasma cells
which produce
antibodies including:
• polyclonal immune globulin
• rheumatoid factor

immune complexes
formed

activates **complement cascade**
(see map)

complement ↑
inflammation and
acute phase reactants
such as C-reactive protein

rheumatoid factor (RF) =
IgM antiglobulin formed
against Fc portion of human IgG

RF is present in 70% of
patients with RA
but also other diseases
such as SLE (see map)

chronic inflammation
(see map)

systemic manifestations
include

vasculitis of small and
medium arteries

rheumatoid nodules

systemic symptoms:
• low grade fever
• weight loss
• malaise

pleural disease:
• interstitial fibrosis
• pulmonary nodules
• pneumonitis / pleuritis

Felty's syndrome =
splenomegaly and
pancytopenia

symmetric arthritis
with joint effusions
commonly involving:
• wrist
• ankles
• elbow
• knees
• cervical spine

usually affects small joints of
hands and feet first:
• metacarpophalangeal (MCP)
• proximal interphalangeal (PIP)

joints are red
swollen, warm, and
painful

pain is characterized by:
• worse with movement
• morning stiffness > 1 hour

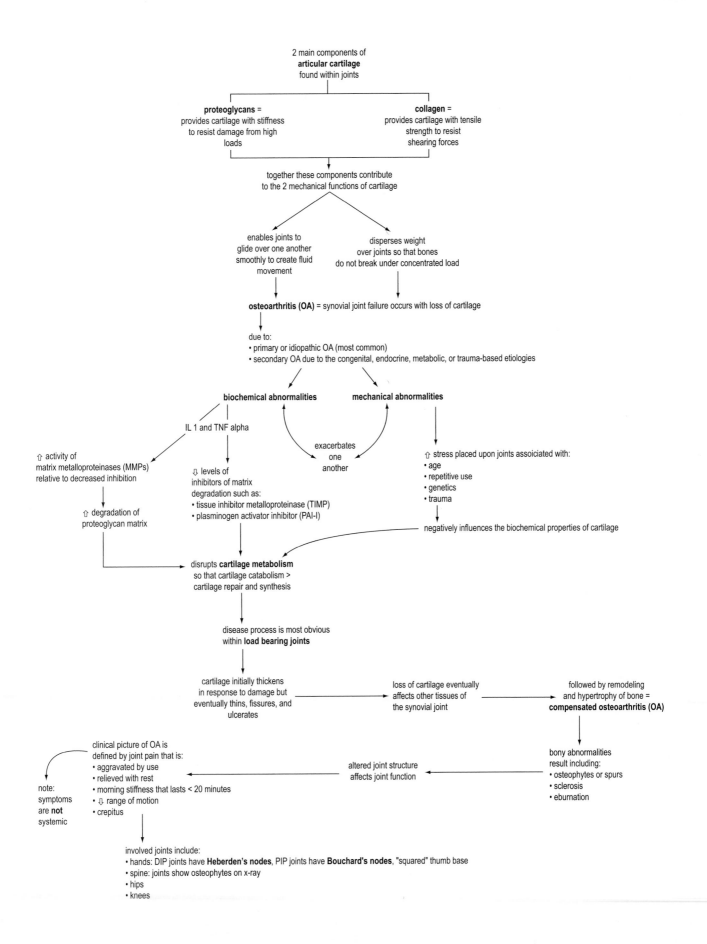

2 main components of
articular cartilage
found within joints

proteoglycans =
provides cartilage with stiffness
to resist damage from high
loads

collagen =
provides cartilage with tensile
strength to resist
shearing forces

together these components contribute
to the 2 mechanical functions of cartilage

enables joints to
glide over one another
smoothly to create fluid
movement

disperses weight
over joints so that bones
do not break under concentrated load

osteoarthritis (OA) = synovial joint failure occurs with loss of cartilage

due to:
• primary or idiopathic OA (most common)
• secondary OA due to the congenital, endocrine, metabolic, or trauma-based etiologies

biochemical abnormalities

mechanical abnormalities

IL 1 and TNF alpha

exacerbates
one
another

⇑ stress placed upon joints assoiciated with:
• age
• repetitive use
• genetics
• trauma

⇑ activity of
matrix metalloproteinases (MMPs)
relative to decreased inhibition

⇩ levels of
inhibitors of matrix
degradation such as:
• tissue inhibitor metalloproteinase (TIMP)
• plasminogen activator inhibitor (PAI-I)

⇑ degradation of
proteoglycan matrix

negatively influences the biochemical properties of cartilage

disrupts **cartilage metabolism**
so that cartilage catabolism >
cartilage repair and synthesis

disease process is most obvious
within **load bearing joints**

cartilage initially thickens
in response to damage but
eventually thins, fissures, and
ulcerates

loss of cartilage eventually
affects other tissues of
the synovial joint

followed by remodeling
and hypertrophy of bone =
compensated osteoarthritis (OA)

clinical picture of OA is
defined by joint pain that is:
• aggravated by use
• relieved with rest
• morning stiffness that lasts < 20 minutes
• ⇩ range of motion
• crepitus

altered joint structure
affects joint function

bony abnormalities
result including:
• osteophytes or spurs
• sclerosis
• eburnation

note:
symptoms
are **not**
systemic

involved joints include:
• hands: DIP joints have **Heberden's nodes**, PIP joints have **Bouchard's nodes**, "squared" thumb base
• spine: joints show osteophytes on x-ray
• hips
• knees

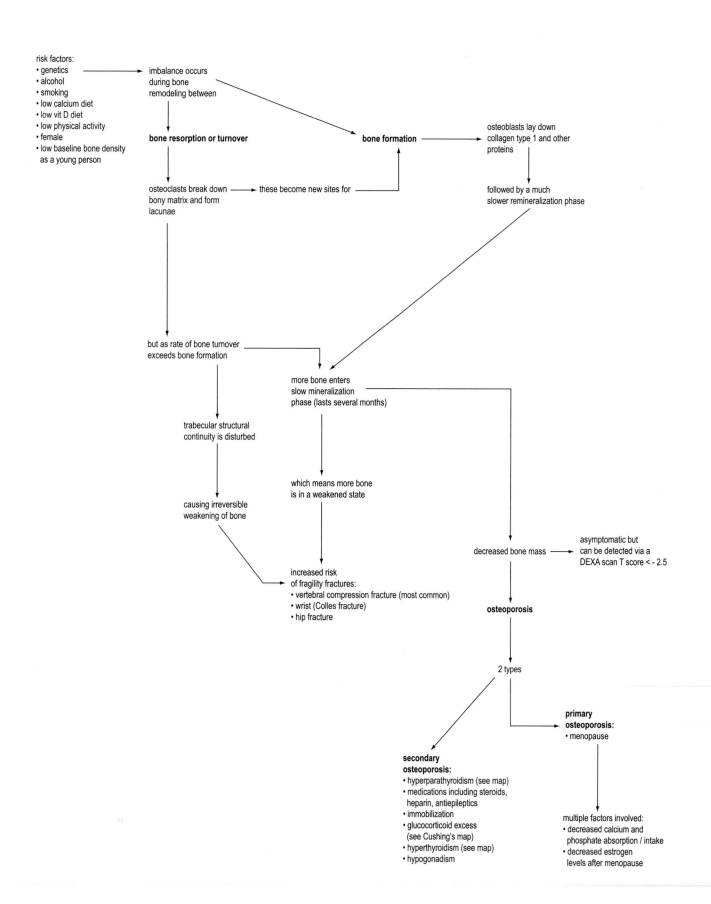

risk factors:
• genetics
• alcohol
• smoking
• low calcium diet
• low vit D diet
• low physical activity
• female
• low baseline bone density
  as a young person

imbalance occurs
during bone
remodeling between

bone resorption or turnover

bone formation

osteoblasts lay down
collagen type 1 and other
proteins

osteoclasts break down
bony matrix and form
lacunae

these become new sites for

followed by a much
slower remineralization phase

but as rate of bone turnover
exceeds bone formation

more bone enters
slow mineralization
phase (lasts several months)

trabecular structural
continuity is disturbed

which means more bone
is in a weakened state

causing irreversible
weakening of bone

decreased bone mass

asymptomatic but
can be detected via a
DEXA scan T score < - 2.5

increased risk
of fragility fractures:
• vertebral compression fracture (most common)
• wrist (Colles fracture)
• hip fracture

osteoporosis

2 types

**secondary
osteoporosis:**
• hyperparathyroidism (see map)
• medications including steroids,
  heparin, antiepileptics
• immobilization
• glucocorticoid excess
  (see Cushing's map)
• hyperthyroidism (see map)
• hypogonadism

**primary
osteoporosis:**
• menopause

multiple factors involved:
• decreased calcium and
  phosphate absorption / intake
• decreased estrogen
  levels after menopause

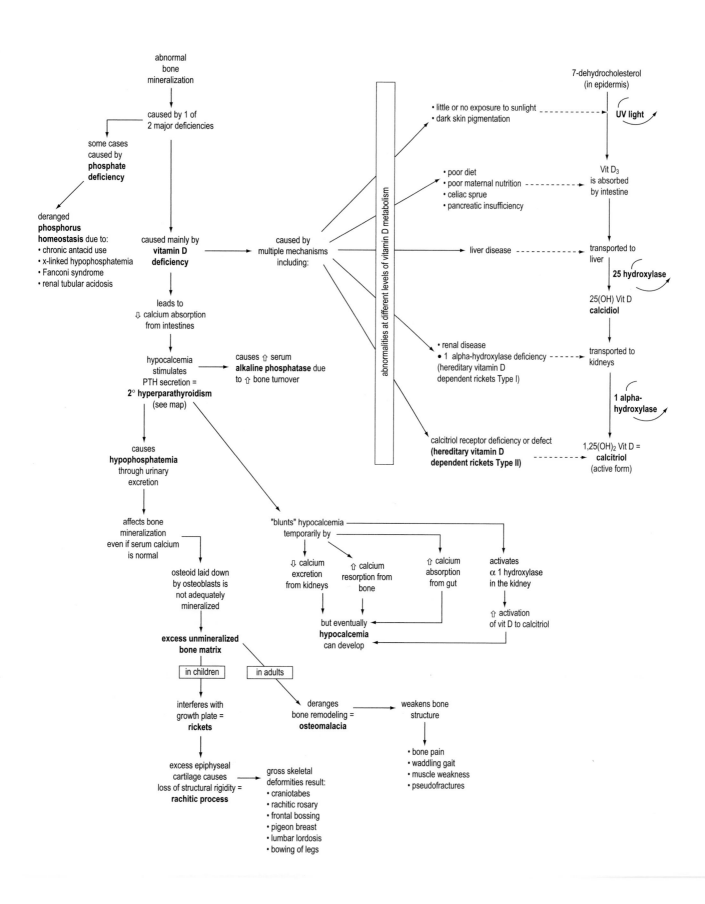

Neurologic Disorders

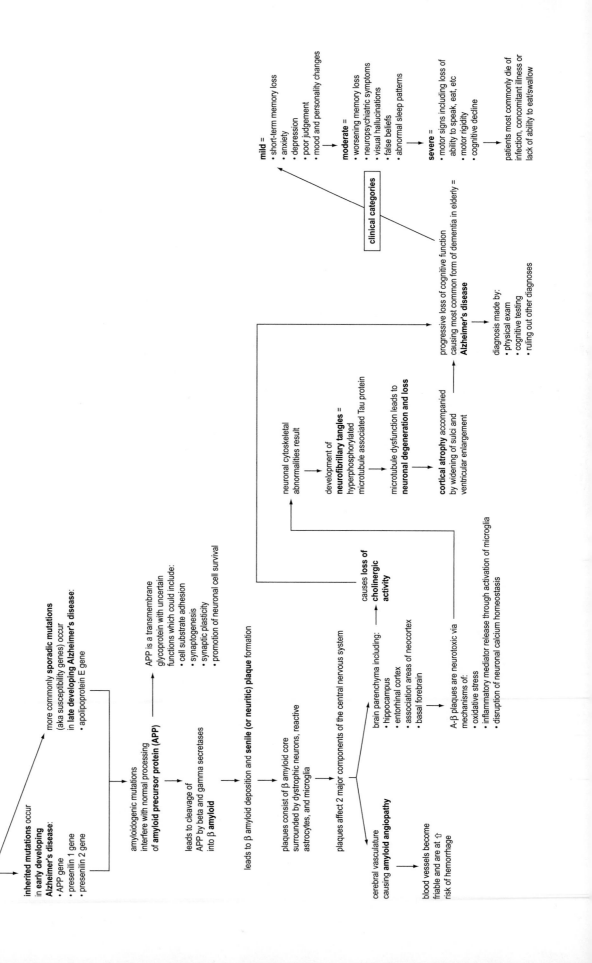

etiology has genetic basis

associations with:
• **trisomy 21**
• traumatic head injury
• high cholesterol
• high homocysteine levels (controversial)

inherited mutations occur in **early developing Alzheimer's disease**:
• APP gene
• presenilin 1 gene
• presenilin 2 gene

more commonly **sporadic mutations** (aka susceptibility genes) occur in **late developing Alzheimer's disease**:
• apolipoprotein E gene

amyloidogenic mutations interfere with normal processing of **amyloid precursor protein (APP)**

APP is a transmembrane glycoprotein with uncertain functions which could include:
• cell substrate adhesion
• synaptogenesis
• synaptic plasticity
• promotion of neuronal cell survival

leads to cleavage of APP by beta and gamma secretases into β **amyloid**

leads to β amyloid deposition and **senile (or neuritic) plaque** formation

plaques consist of β amyloid core surrounded by dystrophic neurons, reactive astrocytes, and microglia

plaques affect 2 major components of the central nervous system

brain parenchyma including:
• hippocampus
• entorhinal cortex
• association areas of neocortex
• basal forebrain

causes **loss of cholinergic activity**

A-β plaques are neurotoxic via mechanisms of:
• oxidative stress
• inflammatory mediator release through activation of microglia
• disruption of neuronal calcium homeostasis

cerebral vasculature causing **amyloid angiopathy**

blood vessels become friable and are at ⇧ risk of hemorrhage

neuronal cytoskeletal abnormalities result

development of **neurofibrillary tangles** = hyperphosphorylated microtubule associated Tau protein

microtubule dysfunction leads to **neuronal degeneration and loss**

cortical atrophy accompanied by widening of sulci and ventricular enlargement

progressive loss of cognitive function causing most common form of dementia in elderly = **Alzheimer's disease**

diagnosis made by:
• physical exam
• cognitive testing
• ruling out other diagnoses

clinical categories

mild =
• short-term memory loss
• anxiety
• depression
• poor judgement
• mood and personality changes

moderate =
• worsening memory loss
• neuropsychiatric symptoms
• visual hallucinations
• false beliefs
• abnormal sleep patterns

severe =
• motor signs including loss of ability to speak, eat, etc
• motor rigidity
• cognitive decline

patients most commonly die of infection, concomitant illness or lack of ability to eat/swallow

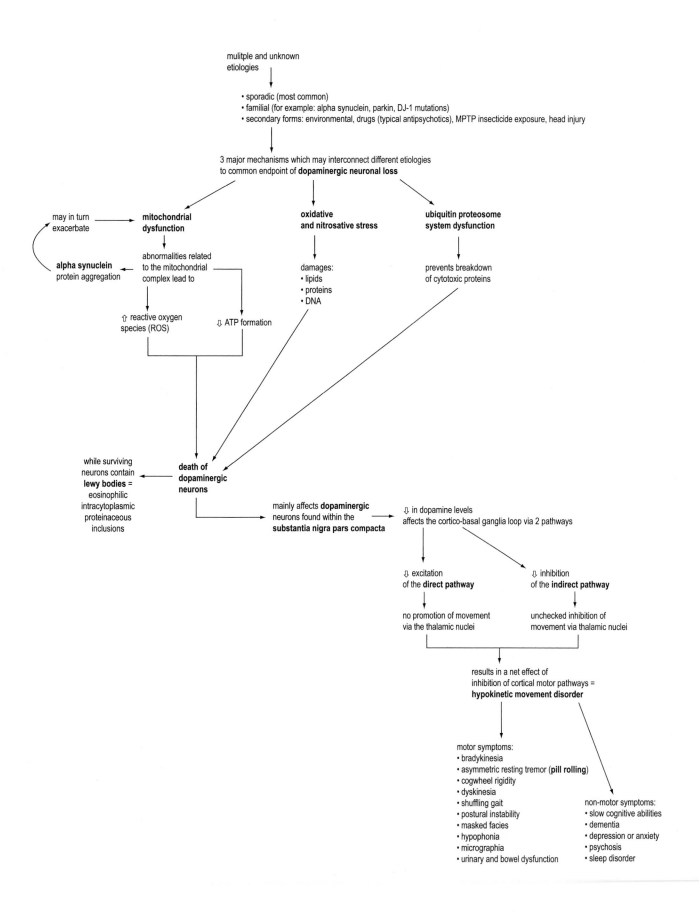

mulitple and unknown
etiologies

- sporadic (most common)
- familial (for example: alpha synuclein, parkin, DJ-1 mutations)
- secondary forms: environmental, drugs (typical antipsychotics), MPTP insecticide exposure, head injury

3 major mechanisms which may interconnect different etiologies
to common endpoint of **dopaminergic neuronal loss**

**mitochondrial
dysfunction**

**oxidative
and nitrosative stress**

**ubiquitin proteosome
system dysfunction**

may in turn
exacerbate

alpha synuclein
protein aggregation

abnormalities related
to the mitochondrial
complex lead to

damages:
- lipids
- proteins
- DNA

prevents breakdown
of cytotoxic proteins

⇑ reactive oxygen
species (ROS)

⇓ ATP formation

while surviving
neurons contain
lewy bodies =
eosinophilic
intracytoplasmic
proteinaceous
inclusions

**death of
dopaminergic
neurons**

mainly affects **dopaminergic**
neurons found within the
substantia nigra pars compacta

⇓ in dopamine levels
affects the cortico-basal ganglia loop via 2 pathways

⇓ excitation
of the **direct pathway**

⇓ inhibition
of the **indirect pathway**

no promotion of movement
via the thalamic nuclei

unchecked inhibition of
movement via thalamic nuclei

results in a net effect of
inhibition of cortical motor pathways =
hypokinetic movement disorder

motor symptoms:
- bradykinesia
- asymmetric resting tremor (**pill rolling**)
- cogwheel rigidity
- dyskinesia
- shuffling gait
- postural instability
- masked facies
- hypophonia
- micrographia
- urinary and bowel dysfunction

non-motor symptoms:
- slow cognitive abilities
- dementia
- depression or anxiety
- psychosis
- sleep disorder

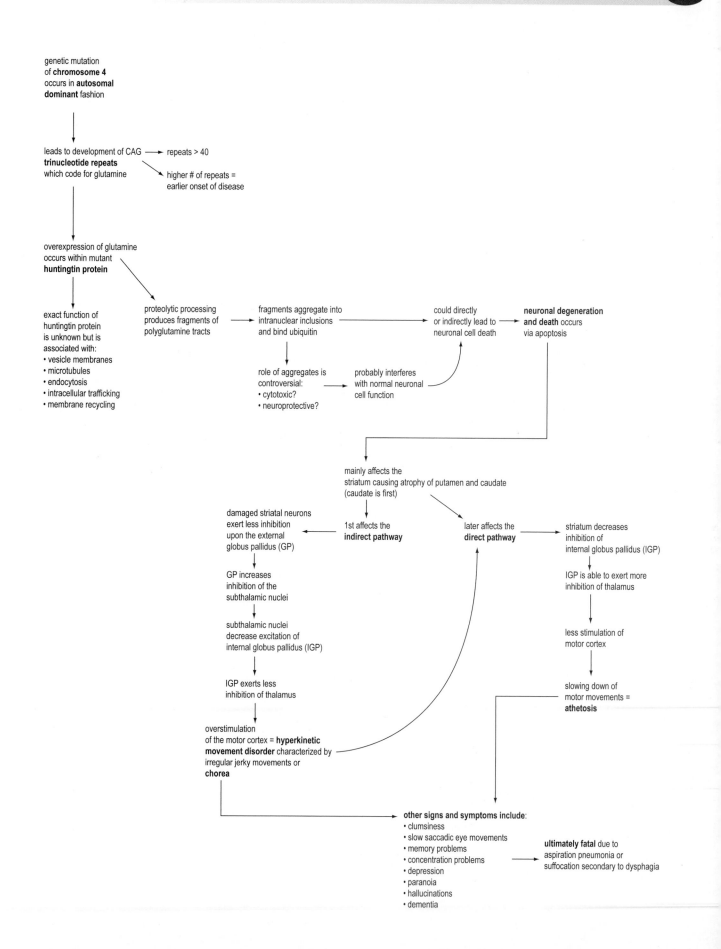

genetic mutation
of **chromosome 4**
occurs in **autosomal
dominant** fashion

leads to development of CAG ⟶ repeats > 40
trinucleotide repeats
which code for glutamine ⟶ higher # of repeats =
earlier onset of disease

overexpression of glutamine
occurs within mutant
huntingtin protein

exact function of
huntingtin protein
is unknown but is
associated with:
• vesicle membranes
• microtubules
• endocytosis
• intracellular trafficking
• membrane recycling

proteolytic processing
produces fragments of
polyglutamine tracts

fragments aggregate into
intranuclear inclusions
and bind ubiquitin

could directly
or indirectly lead to
neuronal cell death

**neuronal degeneration
and death** occurs
via apoptosis

role of aggregates is
controversial:
• cytotoxic?
• neuroprotective?

probably interferes
with normal neuronal
cell function

mainly affects the
striatum causing atrophy of putamen and caudate
(caudate is first)

damaged striatal neurons
exert less inhibition
upon the external
globus pallidus (GP)

1st affects the
indirect pathway

later affects the
direct pathway

striatum decreases
inhibition of
internal globus pallidus (IGP)

GP increases
inhibition of the
subthalamic nuclei

IGP is able to exert more
inhibition of thalamus

subthalamic nuclei
decrease excitation of
internal globus pallidus (IGP)

less stimulation of
motor cortex

IGP exerts less
inhibition of thalamus

slowing down of
motor movements =
athetosis

overstimulation
of the motor cortex = **hyperkinetic
movement disorder** characterized by
irregular jerky movements or
chorea

other signs and symptoms include:
• clumsiness
• slow saccadic eye movements
• memory problems
• concentration problems
• depression
• paranoia
• hallucinations
• dementia

ultimately fatal due to
aspiration pneumonia or
suffocation secondary to dysphagia

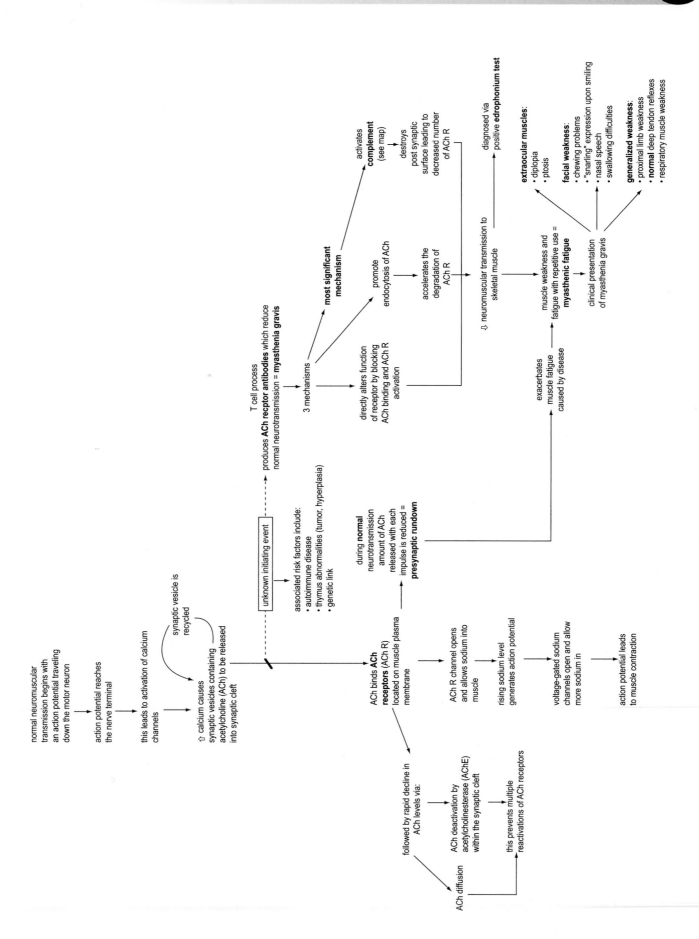

normal neuromuscular transmission begins with an action potential traveling down the motor neuron

action potential reaches the nerve terminal

this leads to activation of calcium channels

synaptic vesicle is recycled

⇧ calcium causes synaptic vesicles containing acetylcholine (ACh) to be released into synaptic cleft

ACh binds ACh receptors (ACh R) located on muscle plasma membrane

ACh R channel opens and allows sodium into muscle

rising sodium level generates action potential

voltage-gated sodium channels open and allow more sodium in

action potential leads to muscle contraction

followed by rapid decline in ACh levels via:

ACh deactivation by acetylcholinesterase (AChE) within the synaptic cleft

this prevents multiple reactivations of ACh receptors

ACh diffusion

unknown initiating event

T cell process

associated risk factors include:
• autoimmune disease
• thymus abnormalities (tumor, hyperplasia)
• genetic link

during **normal** neurotransmission amount of ACh released with each impulse is reduced = **presynaptic rundown**

produces **ACh receptor antibodies** which reduce normal neurotransmission = **myasthenia gravis**

3 mechanisms

activates **complement** (see map)

most significant mechanism

promote endocytosis of ACh

directly alters function of receptor by blocking ACh binding and ACh R activation

destroys post synaptic surface leading to decreased number of ACh R

accelerates the degradation of ACh R

⇩ neuromuscular transmission to skeletal muscle

muscle weakness and fatigue with repetitive use = **myasthenic fatigue**

exacerbates muscle fatigue caused by disease

clinical presentation of myasthenia gravis

diagnosed via positive **edrophonium test**

extraocular muscles:
• diplopia
• ptosis

facial weakness:
• chewing problems
• "snarling" expression upon smiling
• nasal speech
• swallowing difficulties

generalized weakness:
• proximal limb weakness
• **normal** deep tendon reflexes
• respiratory muscle weakness

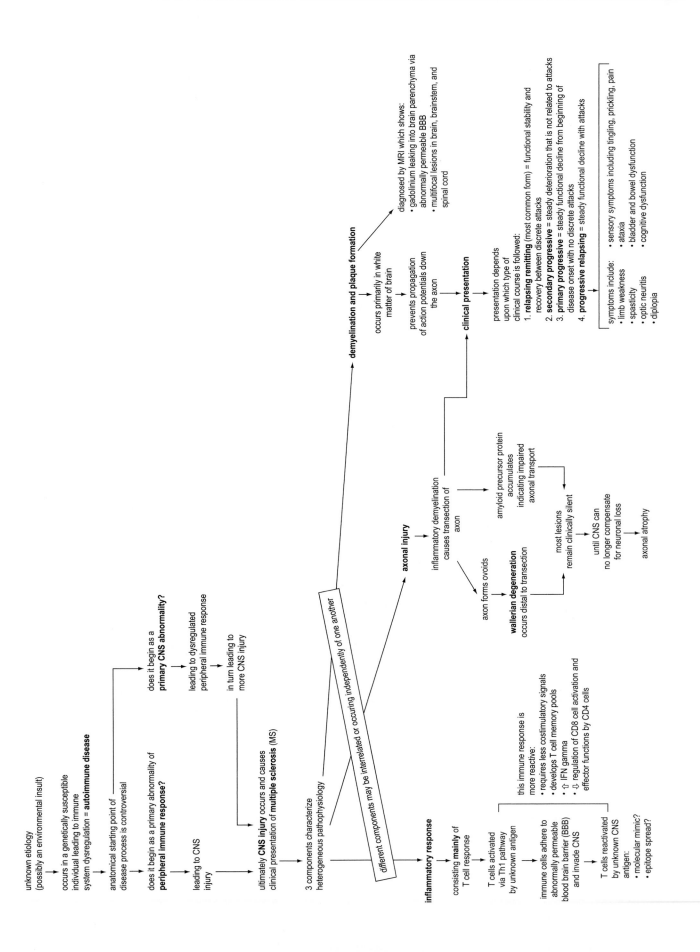

unknown etiology
(possibly an environmental insult)

occurs in a genetically susceptible
individual leading to immune
system dysregulation = **autoimmune disease**

anatomical starting point of
disease process is controversial

does it begin as a primary abnormality of
peripheral immune response?

leading to CNS
injury

does it begin as a
primary CNS abnormality?

leading to dysregulated
peripheral immune response

in turn leading to
more CNS injury

ultimately **CNS injury** occurs and causes
clinical presentation of **multiple sclerosis** (MS)

3 components characterize
heterogeneous pathophysiology

different components may be interrelated or occuring independently of one another

inflammatory response

consisting **mainly** of
T cell response

T cells activated
via Th1 pathway
by unknown antigen

immune cells adhere to
abnormally permeable
blood brain barrier (BBB)
and invade CNS

T cells reactivated
by unknown CNS
antigen:
• molecular mimic?
• epitope spread?

this immune response is
more reactive:
• requires less costimulatory signals
• develops T cell memory pools
• ⇧ IFN gamma
• ⇩ regulation of CD8 cell activation and
  effector functions by CD4 cells

axonal injury

inflammatory demyelination
causes transection of
axon

amyloid precursor protein
accumulates
indicating impaired
axonal transport

axon forms ovoids

wallerian degeneration
occurs distal to transection

most lesions
remain clinically silent

until CNS can
no longer compensate
for neuronal loss

axonal atrophy

demyelination and plaque formation

occurs primarily in white
matter of brain

prevents propagation
of action potentials down
the axon

diagnosed by MRI which shows:
• gadolinium leaking into brain parenchyma via
  abnormally permeable BBB
• multifocal lesions in brain, brainstem, and
  spinal cord

clinical presentation

presentation depends
upon which type of
clinical course is followed:
1. **relapsing remitting** (most common form) = functional stability and
   recovery between discrete attacks
2. **secondary progressive** = steady deterioration that is not related to attacks
3. **primary progressive** = steady functional decline from beginning of
   disease onset with no discrete attacks
4. **progressive relapsing** = steady functional decline with attacks

symptoms include:
• limb weakness
• spasticity
• optic neuritis
• diplopia

• sensory symptoms including tingling, prickling, pain
• ataxia
• bladder and bowel dysfunction
• cognitive dysfunction

multiple mechanisms believed to cause different types of seizures and epileptic syndromes

abnormalities occur at 2 basic levels of central nervous system

level of individual neuron

level of neuronal circuits

abnormalities with neurotransmission:
• ⇩ GABA inhibition
• ⇧ post synaptic excitation
• ⇧ burst frequency of AP
• kindling

abnormalities with extracellular environment:
• ⇧ extracellular K⁺
• altered ion channel function
• glial cell abnormalities
• altered intra- and extracellular ion concentrations

abnormalities with neuronal morphology:
• extracellular space
• mossy fiber sprouting
• gap junctions
• sclerosis
• gliosis
• plasticity
• cortical malformations

contributes to neuronal network abnormality

alters the way neurons communicate with one another creating 2 major components of **epileptogenesis**

hyperexcitability: neurons are more likely to propogate action potentials inappropriately

hypersynchronicity: excitation is more likely to activate and involve neighboring neurons and circuits inappropriately

seizure = repetitive, excessive, and sustained neuronal discharge

recurrent seizures = **epilepsy**

if seizure lasts > 30 minutes = **status epilepticus**

epilepsy syndromes are divided into 2 major categories

partial or focal
one or more localized foci in **one** hemisphere

2 subdivisions of partial seizures based on level of consciousness

simple partial seizures =
• consciousness is preserved
• Jacksonian march

complex partial seizures =
• altered consciousness
• staring
• automatisms such as lip smacking and chewing
• postictal confusion

partial seizures can progress to secondarily generalized seizures

generalized
seizure activity begins in **both** hemispheres at the same time

tonic clonic or grand mal (most common):
• tonic phase = stiffening, fall, cry, legs extended
• clonic phase = jerking of extremities
• drooling, foaming, biting of tongue / cheek / lip
• bowel or bladder incontinence
• postictal confusion or lethargy
• generalized polyspikes on EEG

myoclonic seizures:
• brief shock like jerk of muscle or muscle group
• poly spike and slow wave discharge on EEG

clonic seizures:
several myoclonic seizures occuring in rapid succession

atonic seizures:
• sudden loss of postural tone

tonic seizures:
• flex at waist and neck
• abduction flexion/extension of upper extremities
• usually occur during sleep

absence or **petit mal:**
• staring with impaired awareness or responsiveness
• no postictal confusion
• usually children
• 3 Hz spike-wave discharge on EEG

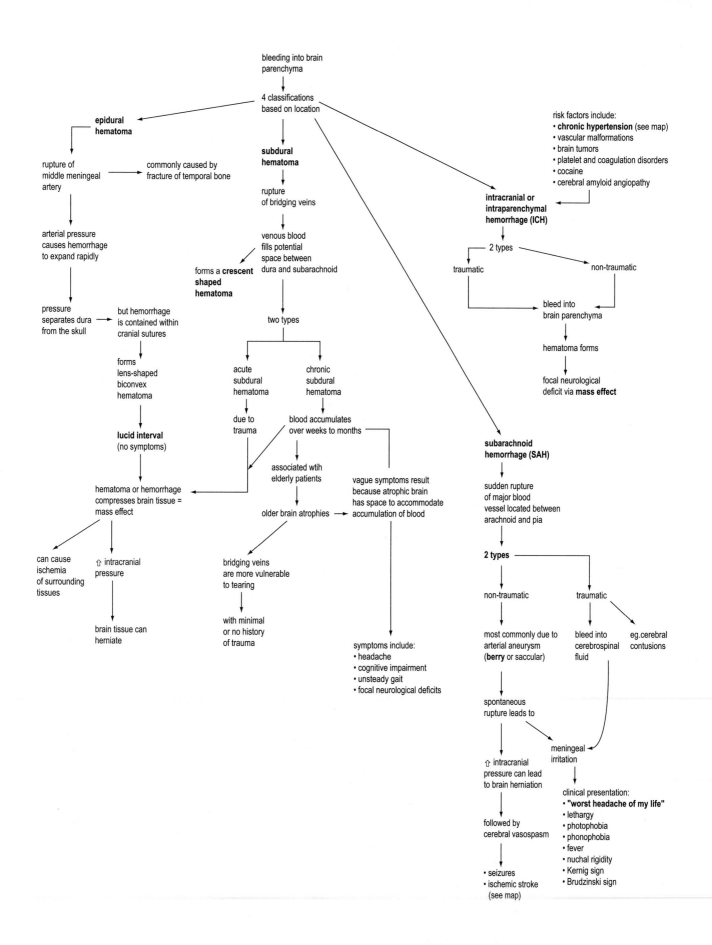

bleeding into brain parenchyma

4 classifications based on location

epidural hematoma

rupture of middle meningeal artery → commonly caused by fracture of temporal bone

arterial pressure causes hemorrhage to expand rapidly

pressure separates dura from the skull → but hemorrhage is contained within cranial sutures

forms lens-shaped biconvex hematoma

lucid interval (no symptoms)

hematoma or hemorrhage compresses brain tissue = mass effect

can cause ischemia of surrounding tissues

⇧ intracranial pressure

brain tissue can herniate

subdural hematoma

rupture of bridging veins

venous blood fills potential space between dura and subarachnoid

forms a **crescent shaped hematoma**

two types

acute subdural hematoma

chronic subdural hematoma

due to trauma

blood accumulates over weeks to months

associated wtih elderly patients

older brain atrophies → vague symptoms result because atrophic brain has space to accommodate accumulation of blood

bridging veins are more vulnerable to tearing

with minimal or no history of trauma

symptoms include:
• headache
• cognitive impairment
• unsteady gait
• focal neurological deficits

risk factors include:
• **chronic hypertension** (see map)
• vascular malformations
• brain tumors
• platelet and coagulation disorders
• cocaine
• cerebral amyloid angiopathy

intracranial or intraparenchymal hemorrhage (ICH)

2 types

traumatic

non-traumatic

bleed into brain parenchyma

hematoma forms

focal neurological deficit via **mass effect**

subarachnoid hemorrhage (SAH)

sudden rupture of major blood vessel located between arachnoid and pia

2 types

non-traumatic

traumatic

most commonly due to arterial aneurysm (**berry** or saccular)

bleed into cerebrospinal fluid

eg.cerebral contusions

spontaneous rupture leads to

meningeal irritation

⇧ intracranial pressure can lead to brain herniation

followed by cerebral vasospasm

• seizures
• ischemic stroke (see map)

clinical presentation:
• **"worst headache of my life"**
• lethargy
• photophobia
• phonophobia
• fever
• nuchal rigidity
• Kernig sign
• Brudzinski sign

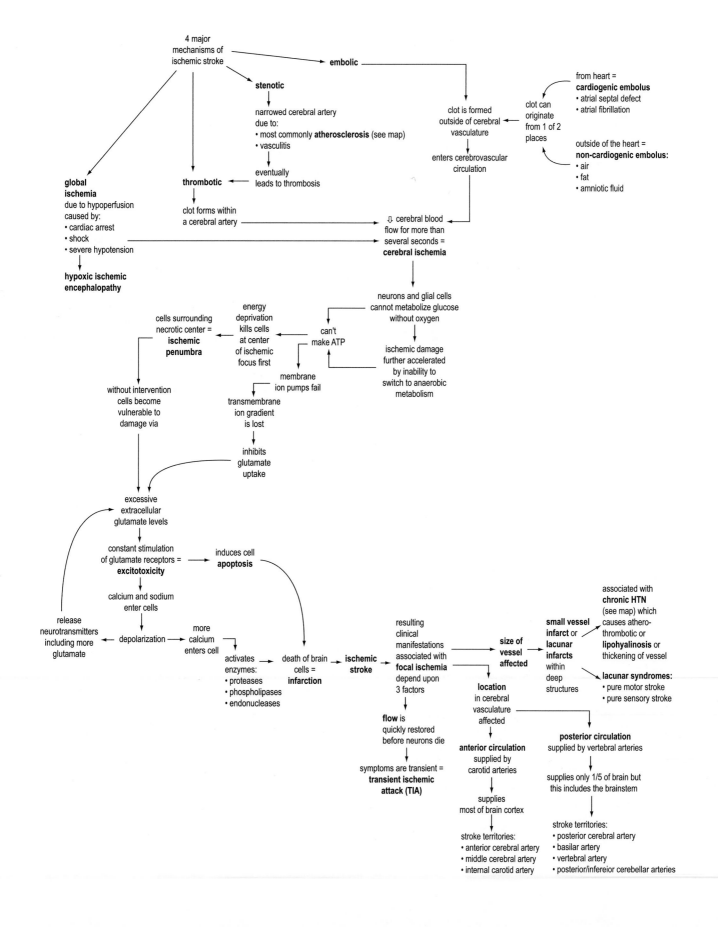

4 major
mechanisms of
ischemic stroke

embolic

stenotic

narrowed cerebral artery
due to:
• most commonly **atherosclerosis** (see map)
• vasculitis

eventually
leads to thrombosis

clot is formed
outside of cerebral
vasculature

enters cerebrovascular
circulation

clot can
originate
from 1 of 2
places

from heart =
cardiogenic embolus
• atrial septal defect
• atrial fibrillation

outside of the heart =
non-cardiogenic embolus:
• air
• fat
• amniotic fluid

**global
ischemia**
due to hypoperfusion
caused by:
• cardiac arrest
• shock
• severe hypotension

thrombotic

clot forms within
a cerebral artery

⇓ cerebral blood
flow for more than
several seconds =
cerebral ischemia

**hypoxic ischemic
encephalopathy**

neurons and glial cells
cannot metabolize glucose
without oxygen

energy
deprivation
kills cells
at center
of ischemic
focus first

can't
make ATP

ischemic damage
further accelerated
by inability to
switch to anaerobic
metabolism

cells surrounding
necrotic center =
**ischemic
penumbra**

membrane
ion pumps fail

without intervention
cells become
vulnerable to
damage via

transmembrane
ion gradient
is lost

inhibits
glutamate
uptake

excessive
extracellular
glutamate levels

constant stimulation
of glutamate receptors =
excitotoxicity

induces cell
apoptosis

calcium and sodium
enter cells

release
neurotransmitters
including more
glutamate

depolarization

more
calcium
enters cell

activates
enzymes:
• proteases
• phospholipases
• endonucleases

death of brain
cells =
infarction

**ischemic
stroke**

resulting
clinical
manifestations
associated with
focal ischemia
depend upon
3 factors

**size of
vessel
affected**

**small vessel
infarct** or
**lacunar
infarcts**
within
deep
structures

associated with
chronic HTN
(see map) which
causes athero-
thrombotic or
lipohyalinosis or
thickening of vessel

lacunar syndromes:
• pure motor stroke
• pure sensory stroke

flow is
quickly restored
before neurons die

symptoms are transient =
**transient ischemic
attack (TIA)**

location
in cerebral
vasculature
affected

anterior circulation
supplied by
carotid arteries

supplies
most of brain cortex

stroke territories:
• anterior cerebral artery
• middle cerebral artery
• internal carotid artery

posterior circulation
supplied by vertebral arteries

supplies only 1/5 of brain but
this includes the brainstem

stroke territories:
• posterior cerebral artery
• basilar artery
• vertebral artery
• posterior/infereior cerebellar arteries

Female Reproductive System Disorders

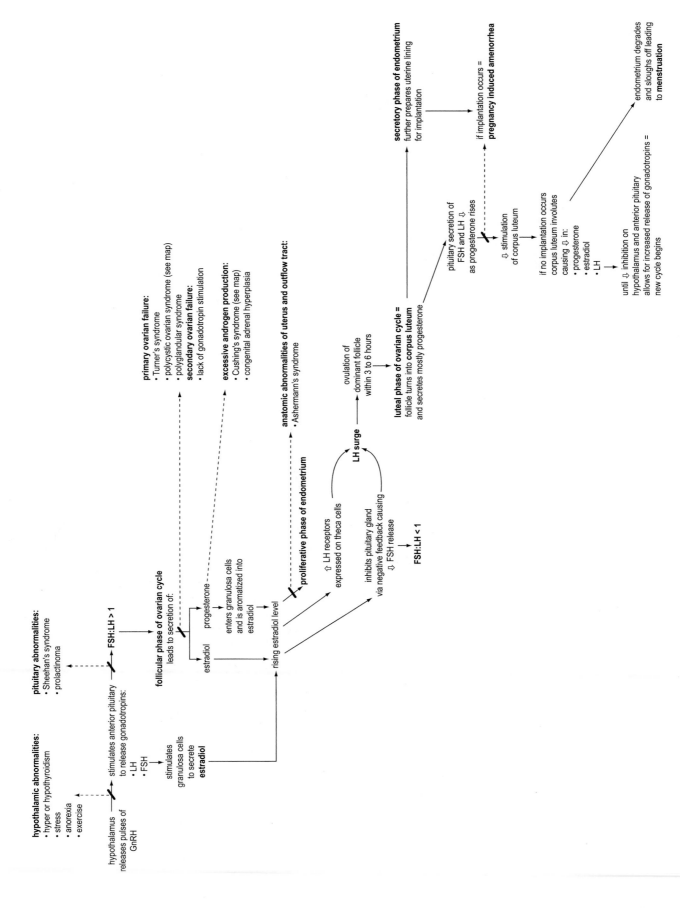

hypothalamic abnormalities:
• hyper or hypothyroidism
• stress
• anorexia
• exercise

hypothalamus releases pulses of GnRH

stimulates anterior pituitary to release gonadotropins:
• LH
• FSH

stimulates granulosa cells to secrete **estradiol**

pituitary abnormalities:
• Sheehan's syndrome
• prolactinoma

FSH:LH > 1

follicular phase of ovarian cycle
leads to secretion of:

estradiol

progesterone

enters granulosa cells and is aromatized into estradiol

rising estradiol level

primary ovarian failure:
• Turner's syndrome
• polycystic ovarian syndrome (see map)
• polyglandular syndrome
secondary ovarian failure:
• lack of gonadotropin stimulation

excessive androgen production:
• Cushing's syndrome (see map)
• congenital adrenal hyperplasia

anatomic abnormalities of uterus and outflow tract:
• Ashermann's syndrome

proliferative phase of endometrium

⇑ LH receptors expressed on theca cells

inhibits pituitary gland via negative feedback causing ⇓ FSH release

FSH:LH < 1

LH surge

ovulation of dominant follicle within 3 to 6 hours

luteal phase of ovarian cycle =
follicle turns into **corpus luteum**
and secretes mostly progesterone

secretory phase of endometrium
further prepares uterine lining for implantation

pituitary secretion of FSH and LH ⇓ as progesterone rises

⇓ stimulation of corpus luteum

if implantation occurs = **pregnancy induced amenorrhea**

if no implantation occurs corpus luteum involutes causing ⇓ in:
• progesterone
• estradiol
• LH

until ⇓ inhibition on hypothalamus and anterior pituitary allows for increased release of gonadotropins = new cycle begins

endometrium degrades and sloughs off leading to **menstruation**

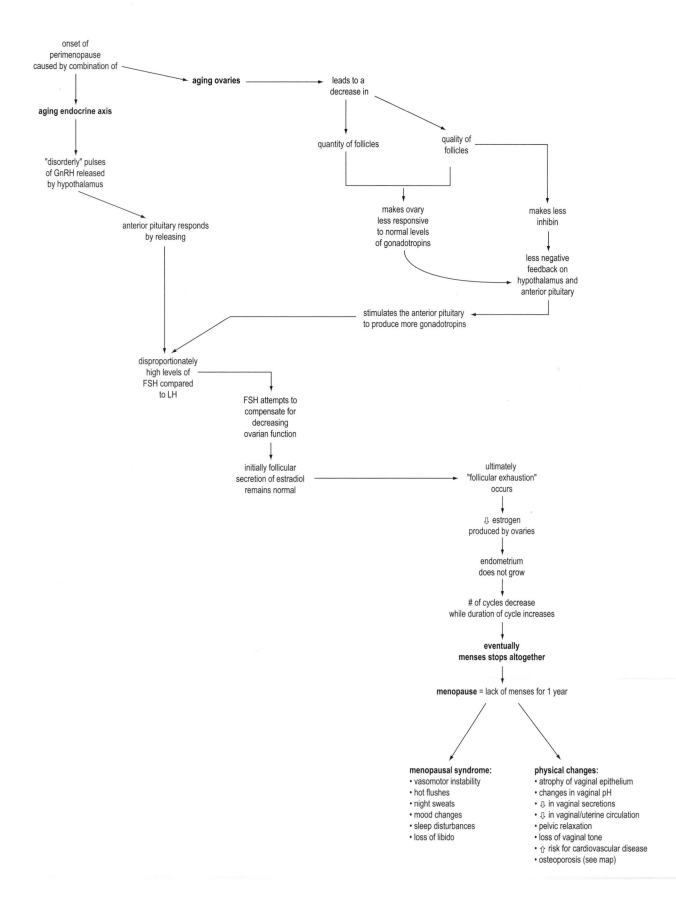

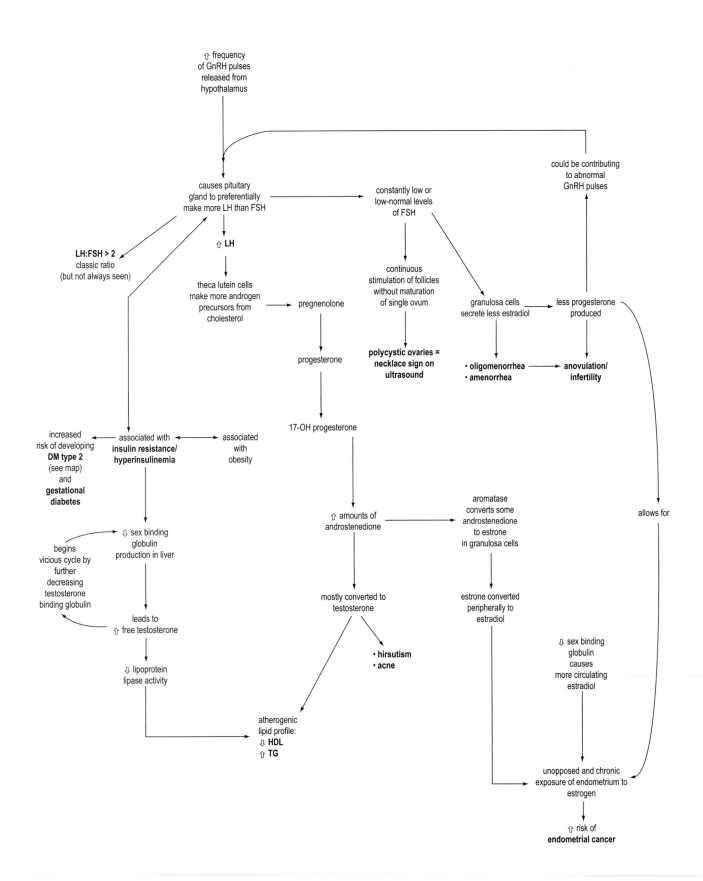

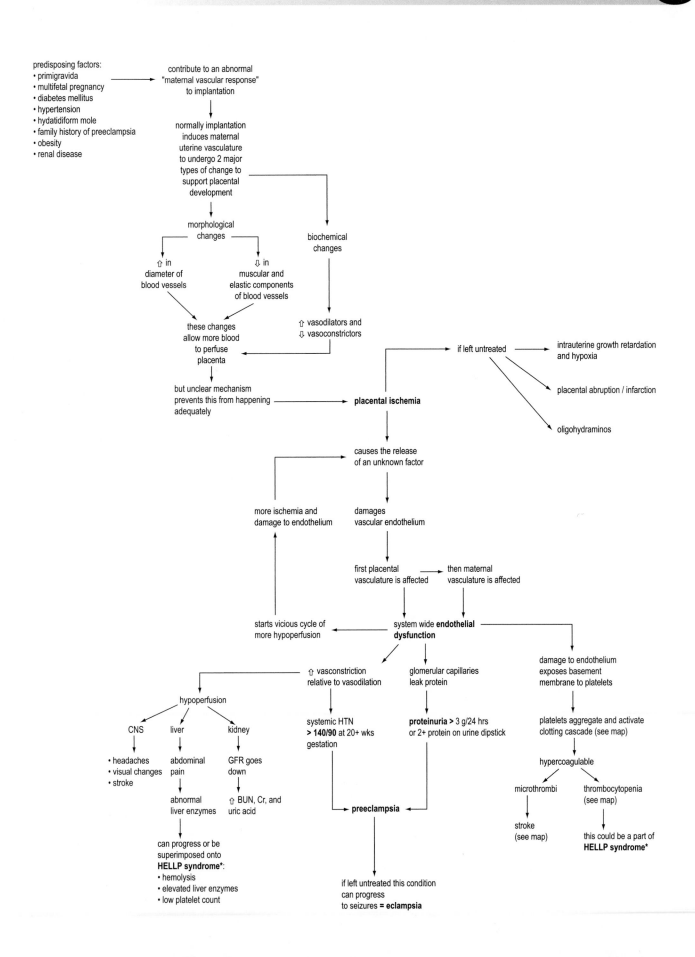

predisposing factors:
• primigravida
• multifetal pregnancy
• diabetes mellitus
• hypertension
• hydatidiform mole
• family history of preeclampsia
• obesity
• renal disease

contribute to an abnormal "maternal vascular response" to implantation

normally implantation induces maternal uterine vasculature to undergo 2 major types of change to support placental development

morphological changes

biochemical changes

⇧ in diameter of blood vessels

⇩ in muscular and elastic components of blood vessels

these changes allow more blood to perfuse placenta

⇧ vasodilators and ⇩ vasoconstrictors

but unclear mechanism prevents this from happening adequately

placental ischemia

if left untreated

intrauterine growth retardation and hypoxia

placental abruption / infarction

oligohydraminos

causes the release of an unknown factor

more ischemia and damage to endothelium

damages vascular endothelium

first placental vasculature is affected

then maternal vasculature is affected

starts vicious cycle of more hypoperfusion

system wide **endothelial dysfunction**

⇧ vasconstriction relative to vasodilation

glomerular capillaries leak protein

damage to endothelium exposes basement membrane to platelets

hypoperfusion

systemic HTN **> 140/90** at 20+ wks gestation

proteinuria > 3 g/24 hrs or 2+ protein on urine dipstick

platelets aggregate and activate clotting cascade (see map)

CNS

liver

kidney

hypercoagulable

• headaches
• visual changes
• stroke

abdominal pain

GFR goes down

microthrombi

thrombocytopenia (see map)

abnormal liver enzymes

⇧ BUN, Cr, and uric acid

preeclampsia

stroke (see map)

this could be a part of **HELLP syndrome***

can progress or be superimposed onto **HELLP syndrome***:
• hemolysis
• elevated liver enzymes
• low platelet count

if left untreated this condition can progress to seizures **= eclampsia**

Normal blood (B), plasma (P), or serum (S) values

	Fluid	Reference Range	System International Reference Range
Alanine aminotransferase (ALT)	S	8–20 U/L	0.13–0.33 kat/L
Aldosterone, with normal sodium intake of 100–200 mEq/day	S	Supine: <16 ng/dL Upright: 4–31 ng/dL	<444 pmol/L 111–860 pmol/L
Arginine vasopressin	P	1.0–13.3 pg/mL	1.0–13.3 ng/L
Aspartate aminotransferase (AST)	S	9–40 U/L	0.15–0.67 kat/L
Bicarbonate, arterial	P	22–26 mEq/L	22–26 mmol/L
Bilirubin, total	S	0.1–1.0 mg/dL	2–17 mol/L
Calcium	S	8.4–10.2 mg/dL	2.1–2.6 mmol/L
Carbon dioxide (PCO_2), arterial	B	35–45 mm Hg	4.7–6.0 kPa
Chloride	P, S	95–105 mEq/L	95–105 mmol/L
Cholesterol, recommended	S	<200 mg/dL	<5.2 mmol/L
Cortisol	S	0800 h: 5–23 g/dL 1600 h: 3–15 g/dL 2000 h: <50% of 0800 h value	138–635 nmol/L 82–413 nmol/L <0.50 of 0800 h value
Creatine kinase	S	Female: 10–70 U/L Male: 25–90 U/L	0.17–1.17 kat/L 0.42–1.50 kat/L
Creatinine	S	0.6–1.2 mg/dL	53–106 mol/L
1,25-Dihydroxyvitamin D	S	16–42 pg/mL	38–101 pmol/L
25-Hydroxyvitamin D	S	8–80 ng/mL	20–200 nmol/L

Estradiol	P, S	Female
		  Prepubertal: <20 pg/mL
		  Premenopausal adult:
		    23–361 pg/mL
		  Postmenopausal adult:
		    <30 pg/mL
		Male: <50 pg/mL
			<73 pmol/L
			
			84–1325 pmol/L
			
			<110 pmol/L
			<184 pmol/L

Ferritin	S	Male: 15–200 ng/mL Female: 12–150 ng/mL	15–200 g/L 12–150 g/L

Follicle-stimulating hormone	S	Male: 4–25 mIU/mL
		Female:
		  Premenopause: 4–30 mIU/mL
		  Midcycle peak: 10–90 mIU/mL
		  Postmenopause: 40–250 mIU/mL
			4–25 U/L
			
			4–30 U/L
			10–90 U/L
			40–250 U/L

Glucagon	P	50–200 pg/mL	50–200 ng/L
Glucose	S	Fasting: 70–110 mg/dL 2-h postprandial: <140 mg/dL	3.9–6.1 mmol/L <7.8 mmol/L

	Fluid	Reference Range	System International Reference Range
Growth hormone	P	2.0–6.0 ng/mL	2.0–6.0 g/L
HDL cholesterol, as major risk factor	S	<35 mg/dL	<0.91 mmol/L
Insulin	S	0–29 U/mL	0–208 pmol/L
Iron	S	50–170 g/dL	9–30 mol/L
Lactate dehydrogenase	S	100–190 U/L	1.7–3.2 kat/L
LDL cholesterol, desirable	S	<130 mg/dL	<3.36 mmol/L
Luteinizing hormone	S	Male: 6–23 mIU/mL Female 　Follicular phase: 5–30 mIU/mL 　Midcycle: 75–150 mIU/mL 　Postmenopause: 30–200 mIU/mL	6–23 U/L 5–30 U/L 75–150 U/L 30–200 U/L
Magnesium	S	1.5–2.0 mEq/L	0.75–1.0 mmol/L
Osmolality	P, S	275–295 mosm/kg H_2O	275–295 mosm/kg H_2O
Oxygen content, arterial	B	17–21 mL/dL	0.17–0.21 L/L
Oxygen saturation, arterial	B	96–100%	0.96–1.00 mol/mol
Oxygen tension (PO_2), arterial	B	75–100 mm Hg	10.0–13.3 kPa
Parathyroid hormone	P	10–60 pg/mL	10–60 ng/L
pH, arterial	B	7.35–7.45	[H^+] 35–45 nmol/L
Phosphatase, alkaline	S	20–70 U/L	0.33–1.17 kat/L
Phosphorus, inorganic	S	3.0–4.5 mg/dL	1.0–1.5 mmol/L
Potassium	S	3.5–5.0 mEq/L	3.5–5.0 mmol/L
Prolactin	S	Female 　Nonpregnant: 3–30 ng/mL 　Pregnant: 10–209 ng/mL 　Postmenopausal: 2–20 ng/mL Male: 2–18 ng/mL	 3–30 g/L 10–209 g/L 2–20 g/L 2–18 g/L
Proteins 　Total 　Albumin 　Globulin	 S S S	 6.0–7.8 g/dL 3.5–5.5 g/dL 2.3–3.5 g/dL	 60–78 g/L 35–55 g/L 23–35 g/L
Sodium	S	136–145 mEq/L	136–145 mmol/L
Testosterone, total, morning	P	Male: 300–1100 ng/dL Female: 20–90 ng/dL	10.4–38.1 nmol/L 0.7–3.1 nmol/L
Thyroid-stimulating hormone	S	0.5–5.0 U/mL	0.5–5.0 mU/L
Thyroxine (T_4), total	S	5–12 g/dL	64–155 nmol/L
Triglycerides, fasting	S	35–160 mg/dL	0.4–1.8 mmol/L
Triiodothyronine (T_3)	S	115–190 ng/dL	1.8–2.9 nmol/L
Urea nitrogen (BUN)	S	7–18 mg/dL	2.5–6.4 mmol urea/L
Uric acid	S	3.0–8.2 mg/dL	0.18–0.49 mmol/L

Hematologic values

Blood volume	Male: averages 69 mL/kg body weight Female: averages 65 mL/kg body weight	
Plasma volume	Male: 25–43 mL/kg body weight Female: 28–45 mL/kg body weight	0.025–0.043 L/kg body weight 0.028–0.045 L/kg body weight
Erythrocyte count	Male: 4.3–5.9 H 10^6/mm^3 Female: 3.5–5.5 H 10^6/mm^3	4.3–5.9 H 10^{12}/L 3.5–5.5 H 10^{12}/L
Erythrocyte sedimentation rate	Male: 0–15 mm/h Female: 0–20 mm/h	0–15 mm/h 0–20 mm/h
Hematocrit	Male: 41–53% Female: 36–46%	0.41–0.53 0.36–0.46
Hemoglobin, blood	Male: 13.5–17.5 g/dL Female: 12.0–16.0 g/dL	2.09–2.71 mmol/L 1.86–2.48 mmol/L
Hemoglobin A$_{1c}$	#6% of total Hb	#0.06 of total Hb
Leukocyte count and differential		
Leukocyte count	4500–11,000/mm^3	4.5–11.0 H 10^9/L
Segmented neutrophils	45–74%	0.45–0.74
Bands	0–4%	0.00–0.04
Eosinophils	0–7%	0.00–0.07
Basophils	0–2%	0.00–0.02
Lymphocytes	16–45%	0.16–0.45
Monocytes	4–10%	0.04–0.10
Mean corpuscular hemoglobin	25.4–34.6 pg/cell	0.39–0.54 fmol/cell
Mean corpuscular hemoglobin conc.	31–36 g/dL	4.81–5.58 mmol Hb/L
Mean corpuscular volume	80–100 m^3	80–100 fL
Partial thromboplastin time, activated	25–40 seconds	25–40 seconds
Platelet count	150,000–400,000/mm^3	150–400 H 10^9/L
Prothrombin time	11–15 seconds	11–15 seconds
Red cell distribution width	11.5–14.5%	0.115–0.145
Reticulocyte count	0.5–1.5% of red cells	0.005–0.0015

REFERENCES

Acute Inflammation

Kumar V, Abbas AK, Fausto N. *Robbins and Cotran Pathologic Basis of Disease.* 7th ed. Elsevier Saunders; 2005.

Acute Renal Failure

Lameire N. The pathophysiology of acute renal failure. *Crit Care Clin.* 2005;21:197–210.

Lingappa VR. Renal disease. In: McPhee SJ, Lingappa VR, Ganong WF. *Pathophysiology of Disease.* 4th ed. McGraw-Hill; 2003.

Palvesky PM. Acute renal failure. *J Am Soc Nephrol.* 2003; 2(2):41–76.

Addison's Disease

Arit W, Allolio B. Adrenal insufficiency. *Lancet.* 2003;361: 1881–1887.

Cooper MS, Stewart PM. Corticosteroid insufficiency in acutely ill patients. *NEJM.* 2003;348:727–734.

McPhee SJ. Disorders of the adrenal cortex. In: McPhee SJ, Lingappa VR, Ganong WF. *Pathophysiology of Disease.* 4th ed. McGraw-Hill; 2003.

Oelkers W. Adrenal insufficiency. *NEJM.* 1996;335(16): 1206–1212.

Stewart JP. Adrenal cortex and endocrine hypertension. In: Adashi EY, Aiello LP, Arnold A, et al. eds. *Larsen: Williams Textbook of Endocrinology.* 10th ed. Elsevier Saunders; 2003.

Torrey SP. Recognition and management of adrenal emergencies. *Emerg Med Clin N Am.* 2005;23:687–702.

Williams GH, Dluhy RG. Disorders of the adrenal cortex. In: Kasper D, Braunwald E, Fauci A, et al. *Harrison's Principles of Internal Medicine.* 16th ed. McGraw-Hill; 2005.

Alpha Thalassemia

Benz EJ. Hemoglobinopathies. In: Kasper D, Braunwald E, Fauci A, et al. *Harrison's Principles of Internal Medicine.* 16th ed. McGraw-Hill; 2005.

Hoffman R, Benz E, Shattil S, et al. *Hematology: Basic Principles and Practice.* 4th ed. Elsevier Saunders; 2005.

Schrier S. Thalassemia: pathophysiology of red cell changes. *Annu Rev Med.* 1994;45:211–218.

Thalassemia graph: % hemoglobin vs gestational age. From www.thalassemia.com/.Children's Hospital and Research Center, Oakland, CA. October 10, 2006.

Alzheimer's Disease

Bird TD, Miller BL. Alzheimer's disease and other dementias. In: Kasper D, Braunwald E, Fauci A, et al. *Harrison's Principles of Internal Medicine.* 16th ed. McGraw-Hill; 2005.

Blumenfeld H. *Neuroanatomy through Clinical Cases.* Sinauer 2002.

Caselli RJ, Boeve BF. The degenerative dementias. In: Goetz CG. *Textbook of Clinical Neurology.* 2nd ed. Elsevier Saunders; 2003.

Imbimbo B, Lombard J, Pomara N. Pathophysiology of Alzheimer's disease. *Neuroimaging Clin N Am.* 2005;15(4): 767–777.

Martin J. Mechanisms of disease: molecular basis of the neurodegenerative disorders. *NEJM.* 1999;340:1970–1980.

Messing RO. Nervous system disorders. In: McPhee SJ, Lingappa VR, Ganong WF. *Pathophysiology of Disease.* 4th ed. McGraw-Hill; 2003.

Silvestrelli G, Lanari A, Parnetti L, et al. Treatment of Alzheimer's disease: from pharmacology to a better understanding of disease pathophysiology. *Mech Ageing Dev.* 2006;127:148–157.

Amenorrhea

Beckmann C. *Obstetrics and Gynecology.* Lippincott Williams & Wilkins; 2006.

Boron W, Boulpaep E. *Medical Physiology: A Cellular and Molecular Approach.* Elsevier Saunders; 2005.

Lingappa VR. Disorders of the female reproductive tract. In: McPhee SJ, Lingappa VR, Ganong WF. *Pathophysiology of Disease.* 4th ed. McGraw-Hill; 2003.

Anemia of Chronic Disease

Adamson JW. Iron deficiency and other hypoproliferative anemias. In: Kasper D, Braunwald E, Fauci A, et al. eds. *Harrison's Principles of Internal Medicine.* 16th ed. McGraw-Hill; 2005.

Andrews N. Disorders of iron metabolism. *NEJM.* 1999;341: 1986–1995.

Weiss G, Goodnough L. Anemia of chronic disease. *NEJM.* 2005;352:1011–1023.

Acute Respiratory Distress Syndrome

Cheng I, Matthay M. Acute lung injury and the acute respiratory distress syndrome. *Crit Care Clin.* 2003;19:693–712.

Dechert R. The pathophysiology of acute respiratory distress syndrome. *Respir Care Clin.* 2003;9:283–296.

Perina D. Noncardiogenic pulmonary edema. *Emerg Med Clin N Am.* 2003;21:385–393.

Piantadosi C, Schwartz D. The acute respiratory distress syndrome. *Ann Intern Med.* 2004;141:460–470.

Ware L, Matthay M. The acute respiratory distress syndrome. *NEJM.* 2000;342:1334–1349.

Asthma

Boushey Jr. HA, Corry DB, Fahy JV, et al. Asthma. In: Mason R, Murray J, Broaddus V, et al. *Murray and Nadel's Textbook of Respiratory Medicine.* 4th ed. Elsevier Saunders; 2005.

Busse W, Lemanske R. Advances in immunology: Asthma. *NEJM.* 2001;344:350–362.

Prendergast TJ, Ruoss SJ. Pulmonary disease. In: McPhee SJ, Lingappa VR, Ganong WF. *Pathophysiology of Disease.* 4th ed. McGraw-Hill; 2003.

Atherosclerosis

Ganong WF. Cardiovascular disorders: vascular disease. In: McPhee SJ, Lingappa VR, Ganong WF. *Pathophysiology of Disease.* 4th ed. McGraw-Hill; 2003.

Libby P. The pathogenesis of atherosclerosis. In: Kasper D, Braunwald E, Fauci A, et al. ed. *Harrison's Principles of Internal Medicine.* 16th eds. McGraw-Hill; 2005.

Lilly L ed. *Pathophysiology of Heart Disease: A Collaborative Project of Medical Students and Faculty.* 3rd ed. Lippincott Williams & Wilkins; 2003.

Schacter M. The pathogenesis of atherosclerosis. *Int J Cardiol.* 1997;62(Suppl 2):S3–S7.

Schoen FJ. The heart. Kumar V, Abbas AK, Fausto N. *Robbins and Cotran Pathologic Basis of Disease.* 7th ed. Elsevier Saunders; 2005.

Beta Thalassemia

Benz EJ. Hemoglobinopathies. In: Kasper D, Braunwald E, Fauci A, et al. eds. *Harrison's Principles of Internal Medicine.* 16th ed. McGraw-Hill; 2005.

Rund D, Rachmilewitz E. Beta thalassemia. *NEJM.* 2005;353:1135–1146.

Thalassemia graph: % hemoglobin vs. gestational age. From www.thalassemia.com/.Children's Hospital and Research Center, Oakland, CA. Oct 10, 2006.

Thein SL. Pathophysiology of beta thalassemia–a guide to molecular therapies. *Hematology* 2005;2005:31–37.

Cell-Mediated Immunity

Janeway CA, Travers P, Walport M, et al. *Immunobiology: The Immune System in Health and Disease.* 5th ed. Garland Publishers; 2001.

Kindt TJ, Goldsby RA, Osborne BA, et al. *Kuby Immunology.* 6th ed. W.H. Freeman; 2007.

Parham P. *The Immune System.* Garland Publishers; 2000.

Cholelithiasis

Ahmed A, Cheung RC, Keeffe EB. Management of gallstones and their complications. *Am Fam Physician.* 2000;61(6):1673–1680.

Greenberger NJ, Paumgartner G. Diseases of the gallbladder and bile ducts. In: Kasper D, Braunwald E, Fauci A, et al. eds. *Harrison's Principles of Internal Medicine.* 16th ed. McGraw-Hill; 2005.

Horton JD, Bilhartz LE. Gallstone disease and its complications. In: Andrews JM, Angulo P, Anthony T, et al. eds. *Feldman: Sleisenger & Fordtran's Gastrointestinal and Liver Disease.* 7th ed. Elsevier Saunders; 2002.

Lingappa VR. Gastrointestinal disease. In: McPhee SJ, Lingappa VR, Ganong WF. *Pathophysiology of Disease.* 4th ed. McGraw-Hill; 2003.

Chronic Inflammation

Kindt TJ, Goldsby RA, Osborne BA, et al. *Kuby Immunology.* 6th ed. W.H. Freeman; 2007.

Kumar V, Abbas AK, Fausto N. *Robbins and Cotran Pathologic Basis of Disease.* 7th ed. Elsevier Saunders; 2005.

Chronic Renal Failure

Chung RT, Podolsky DK. Cirrhosis and its complications. In: Kasper D, Braunwald E, Fauci A, et al. eds. *Harrison's Principles of Internal Medicine.* 16th ed. McGraw-Hill; 2005.

Skorecki K, Green J Deceased, Brenner BM. Chronic renal failure. In: Kasper D, Braunwald E, Fauci A, et al. eds. *Harrison's Principles of Internal Medicine.* 16th ed. McGraw-Hill; 2005.

Cirrhosis

Lingappa VR. Liver disease. In: McPhee SJ, Lingappa VR, Ganong WF. *Pathophysiology of Disease.* 4th ed. McGraw-Hill; 2003.

Lingappa VR. Renal disease. In: McPhee SJ, Lingappa VR, Ganong WF. *Pathophysiology of Disease.* 4th ed. McGraw-Hill; 2003.

Wong F, Blendis L. New challenge of hepatorenal syndrome: prevention and treatment. *Hepatology.* 2001;34:1242–1251.

Coagulation Cascade

Davie EW, Fujikawa K, Kisiel W. The coagulation cascade: initiation, maintenance, and regulation. *Biochemistry.* 1991;30(43):10363–10370.

Handin RI. Bleeding and thrombosis. In: Kasper D, Braunwald E, Fauci A, et al. eds. *Harrison's Principles of Internal Medicine.* 16th ed. McGraw-Hill; 2005.

Jagneaux T, Taylor DE, Kantrow SP. Coagulation in sepsis. *Am J Med Sci.* 2004;328(4):196–204.

Mitchell RN. Hemodynamic disorders, thromboembolic disease, and shock. In: Kumar V, Abbas AK, Fausto N. *Robbins and Cotran Pathologic Basis of Disease.* 7th ed. Elsevier Saunders; 2005.

Complement Cascade

Janeway CA, Travers P, Walport M, et al. *Immunobiology: The Immune System in Health and Disease.* 5th ed. Garland Publishers; 2001.

Kindt TJ, Goldsby RA, Osborne BA, et al. eds. *Kuby Immunology.* 6th ed. W.H. Freeman; 2007.

Parham P. *The Immune System.* Garland Publishers; 2000.

Congestive Heart Failure

Braunwald E. Heart failure and cor pulmonale. In: Kasper D, Braunwald E, Fauci A, et al. eds. *Harrison's Principles of Internal Medicine.* 16th ed. McGraw-Hill; 2005.

Jessup M, Brozena S. Heart failure. *NEJM.* 2003;348: 2007–2018.

Katz AM. Pathophysiology of heart failure: identifying targets for pharmacotherapy. *Med Clin N Am.* 2003;87:303–316.

Kusumoto F. Cardiovascular disorders: heart disease. In: McPhee SJ, Lingappa VR, Ganong WF. *Pathophysiology of Disease.* 4th ed. McGraw-Hill; 2003.

Mann, DL, Bristow MR. Mechanisms and models in heart failure: the biomechanical model and beyond. *Circulation.* 2005; 111:2837–2849.

Chronic Obstructive Pulmonary Disease

Adams L, Alberg AJ, Albertine KH, et al. *Mason: Murray & Nadel's Textbook of Respiratory Medicine.* 4th ed. Elsevier Saunders; 2005.

Barnes PJ. Chronic obstructive pulmonary disease. *NEJM.* 2000;343:269–280.

Doherty DE. The pathophysiology of airway dysfunction. *Am J Med.* 2004;117 Suppl 12A:11S–23S.

Prendergast TJ, Ruoss SJ. Pulmonary disease. In: McPhee SJ, Lingappa VR, Ganong WF. *Pathophysiology of Disease.* 4th ed. McGraw-Hill; 2003.

Reilly JJ, Silverman EK, Shapiro SD. Chronic obstructive pulmonary disease. In: Kasper D, Braunwald E, Fauci A, et al. eds. *Harrison's Principles of Internal Medicine.* 16th ed. McGraw-Hill; 2005.

Tetly TD. Macrophages and the pathogenesis of COPD. *Chest.* 2002;121:156–159.

Cor Pulmonale

Brunwald E. Heart failure and cor pulmonale. In: Kasper D, Braunwald E, Fauci A, et al. eds. *Harrison's Principles of Internal Medicine.* 16th ed. McGraw-Hill; 2005.

De Marco T, Rapaport E. Cor pulmonale. In: Mason RJ, Murray JF, Broaddus VC, et al. eds. *Murray & Nadel's Textbook of Respiratory Medicine.* 4th ed. Saunders; 2005.

Dyer GS, Fifer MA. Heart failure. In: Lilly LS. ed. *Pathophysiology of Heart Disease: A Collaborative Project of Medical Students and Faculty.* 3rd ed. Lippincott Williams & Wilkins; 2003.

Crohn's Disease

Bamias G, Nyce MR, De La Rue SA, et al. New concepts in the pathophysiology of inflammatory bowel disease. *Ann Intern Med.* 2005;143:895–904.

Friedman S, Blumberg RS. Inflammatory bowel disease. In: Kasper D, Braunwald E, Fauci A, et al. eds. *Harrison's Principles of Internal Medicine.* 16th ed. McGraw-Hill; 2005.

Liu C, Crawford JM. The gastrointestinal system. In: Kumar V, Abbas AK, Fausto N. *Robbins and Cotran Pathologic Basis of Disease.* 7th ed. Elsevier Saunders; 2005.

Podolsky DK. Inflammatory bowel disease. *NEJM.* 2002;347: 417–429.

Cushing's Syndrome

Larsen PR, Kronenberg HM, Melmed S, et al. *Williams Textbook of Endocrinology.* 10th ed. Elsevier Saunders; 2003.

McPhee SJ. Disease of the adrenal cortex. In: McPhee SJ, Lingappa VR, Ganong WF. *Pathophysiology of Disease.* 4th ed. McGraw-Hill; 2003.

Newell-Price J, Bertagna X, Grossman AB, et al. Cushing's syndrome. *Lancet.* 2006;367:1605–1617.

Raff H, Findling JW. A physiologic approach to diagnosis of Cushing's syndrome. *Ann Intern Med.* 2003;138:980–991.

Williams GH, Dluhy RG. Disorders of the adrenal cortex. In: Kasper D, Braunwald E, Fauci A, et al. eds. *Harrison's Principles of Internal Medicine.* 16th ed. McGraw-Hill; 2005.

Cystic Fibrosis

Boucher RC, Knowles MR, Yankaskas JR. Cystic fibrosis. In: Mason RJ, Murray JF, Broaddus VC, et al. eds. *Mason: Murray & Nadel's Textbook of Respiratory Medicine.* 4th ed. Saunders; 2005.

Boucher RC. Cystic fibrosis. In: Kasper D, Braunwald E, Fauci A, et al. *Harrison's Principles of Internal Medicine.* 16th ed. McGraw-Hill; 2005.

Gibson RL, Burns JL, Ramsey BW. Pathophysiology and management of infections in cystic fibrosis. *Am J Resp Crit Care Med.* 2003;168:918–951.

Maitra A, Kumar V. Diseases of infancy and childhood. In: Kumar V, Abbas AK, Fausto N. *Robbins and Cotran Pathologic Basis of Disease,* 7th ed. Elsevier Saunders, 2005.

Whitcomb DC. Hereditary and childhood disorders of the pancreas, including cystic fibrosis. In: Tschumy WO, Friedman LS, Sleisenger MH et al. eds. *Feldman: Sleisenger & Fordtran's Gastrointestinal and Liver Disease.* 7th ed. Saunders; 2002.

Diabetes Insipidus

Boron WF, Boulpaep EL. Medical physiology: a cellular and molecular approach. 1st ed. Elsevier Saunders; 2003.

Lingappa VR. Disorders of the hypothalamus and pituitary gland. In: McPhee SJ, Lingappa VR, Ganong WF. *Pathophysiology of Disease.* 4th ed. McGraw-Hill; 2003.

Morello JP, Bichet DG. Nephrogenic diabetes insipidus. *Annu Rev Physiol.* 2001;63:607–630.

Robertson GL. Diabetes insipidus. In: Kasper D, Braunwald E, Fauci A, et al. eds. *Harrison's Principles of Internal Medicine.* 16th ed. McGraw-Hill; 2005.

Sands JM, Bichet DG. Nephrogenic diabetes insipidus. *Ann Intern Med.* 2006;144:186–194.

Diabetes Type 1

Funk JL. Disorders of the endocrine pancreas. In: McPhee SJ, Lingappa VR, Ganong WF. *Pathophysiology of Disease.* 4th ed. McGraw-Hill; 2003.

Powers AC. Diabetes mellitus. In: Kasper D, Braunwald E, Fauci A, et al. eds. *Harrison's Principles of Internal Medicine.* 16th ed. McGraw-Hill; 2005.

Diabetes Type 2

Funk JL. Disorders of the endocrine pancreas. In: McPhee SJ, Lingappa VR, Ganong WF. *Pathophysiology of Disease.* 4th ed. McGraw-Hill; 2003.

Powers AC. Diabetes mellitus. In: Kasper D, Braunwald E, Fauci A, et al. eds. *Harrison's Principles of Internal Medicine.* 16th ed. McGraw-Hill; 2005.

Disseminated Intravascular Coagulation

Aster JC. Red Blood cell and bleeding disorders. In: Kumar V, Abbas AK, Fausto N. *Robbins and Cotran Pathologic Basis of Disease.* 7th ed. Elsevier Saunders; 2005.

Bick RL. Disseminated intravascular coagulation: current concepts of etiology, pathophysiology, diagnosis, and treatment. *Hematol Oncol Clin North Am.* 2003;17(1):149–176.

Handin RI. Disorders of coagulation and thrombosis. In: Kasper D, Braunwald E, Fauci A, et al. eds. *Harrison's Principles of Internal Medicine.* 16th ed. McGraw-Hill; 2005.

Levi M, Cate HT. Disseminated intravascular coagulation. *NEJM.* 1999;341:586–592.

Levi M. Disseminated intravascular coagulation: what's new? *Crti Care Clin,* 2005;21(3):449–467.

Lichtman MA, Beutler E, Williams WJ. In: *Williams Hematology.* 7th ed. McGraw Hill; 2006.

Miller RD, ed. *Miller's Anesthesia.* 6th ed. Elsevier/Churchill Livingstone; 2005.

Zeerleder S, Hack CE, Wuillemin WA. Disseminated intravascular coagulation in sepsis. *Chest.* 2005;128:2864–2875.

Epilepsy

Blumenfeld H. *Neuroanatomy through Clinical Cases.* Sinauer; 2002.

Kapit W, Macey RI, Meisami E. *The Physiology Coloring Book.* 2nd ed. Addison Wesley Longman; 2000.

Najm I, Ying Z, Janigro D. Mechanisms of epileptogenesis. *Neurol Clin.* 2001;19(2):237–250.

Tortora GJ, Grabowski SR. *Principles of Anatomy and Physiology.* 9th ed. Wiley; 2000.

ETOH Hepatitis

Maher JJ. Alcoholic liver disease. In: Feldman M, Friedman LS, Sleisenger MH, eds. In: Sleisenger & Fordtran's Gastrointestinal and Liver Disease: Pathophysiology, Diagnosis, Management. 7th ed. Saunders; 2002.

Mailliard ME, Sorrell MF. Alcoholic liver disease. In: Kasper D, Braunwald E, Fauci A, et al. eds. *Harrison's Principles of Internal Medicine.* 16th ed. McGraw-Hill; 2005.

Sougioultzis S, Dalakas E, Hayes PC, et al. Alcoholic hepatitis: from pathogenesis to treatment. *Curr Med Res Opin.* 2005; 21(9):1337–1346.

Gastroesophageal Reflux Disease

Kahrilas PJ, Pandolfino JE. Gastroesophageal reflux disease and its complications, including Barrett's metaplasia. In: Andrews JM, Angulo P, Anthony T, et al. eds. *Feldman: Sleisenger & Fordtran's Gastrointestinal and Liver Disease.* 7th ed. Elsevier Saunders; 2002.

Kahrilas PJ, Lee TJ. Pathophysiology of gastroesophageal reflux disease. *Thorac Surg Clin.* 2005;15(3):323–333.

Orlando RC. Pathogenesis of reflux esophagitis and Barrett's esophagus. *Med Clin North Am.* 2005;89(2): 219–241.

Tack J. Recent developments in the pathophysiology and therapy of gastroesophageal reflux disease and nonerosive reflux disease. *Curr Opin Gastroenterol.* 2005;21: 454–460.

Glomerulonephritis/Nephritis Syndrome

Alpers CE. The kidney. In: Kumar V, Abbas AK, Fausto N. *Robbins and Cotran Pathologic Basis of Disease.* 7th ed. Elsevier Saunders; 2005.

Hricik DE, Chung-Park M, Sedor JR. Glomerulonephritis. *NEJM.* 1998;339:888–899.

Lau KK. Glomerulonephritis. *Adolesc Med Clin.* 2005;16(1): 67–85.

Gout

Cohen MD. The clinical manifestations of chronic hyperuricemia: focus on gout. Based on proceedings of a symposium on Oct 21, 2004 in San Antonio, TX.

Greidinger EL, Rosen A. Inflammatory rheumatic diseases. In: McPhee SJ, Lingappa VR, Ganong WF. *Pathophysiology of Disease.* 4th ed. McGraw-Hill; 2003.

Reginato AJ. Gout and other crystal arthropathies. In: Kasper D, Braunwald E, Fauci A, et al. eds. *Harrison's Principles of Internal Medicine.* 16th ed. McGraw-Hill; 2005.

Schumacher HR. Pathophysiology of hyperuricemia: the role of uric acid in gout. Based on proceedings of a symposium on Oct 21, 2004 in San Antonio, TX.

Heart Failure (left, right, congestive)

Aurigemma GP, Gaasch WH. Diastolic heart failure. *NEJM.* 2004;351:1097–1105.

Braunwald E. Heart failure and cor pulmonale. In: Kasper D, Braunwald E, Fauci A, et al. *Harrison's Principles of Internal Medicine.* 16th ed. McGraw-Hill; 2005.

Jessup M, Brozena S. Heart failure. *NEJM.* 2003;348: 2007–2018.

Kusumoto F. Cardiovascular disorders: heart disease. In: McPhee SJ, Lingappa VR, Ganong WF. *Pathophysiology of Disease.* 4th ed. McGraw-Hill; 2003.

Lilly LS, ed. *Pathophysiology of Heart Disease: A Collaborative Project of Medical Students and Faculty.* 3rd ed. Lippincott Williams & Wilkins; 2003.

Schoen FJ. The heart. In: Kumar V, Abbas AK, Fausto N. *Robbins and Cotran Pathologic Basis of Disease.* 7th ed. Elsevier Saunders; 2005.

Hemochromatosis

Adams PC. Hemochromatosis. *Clin Liver Disease.* 2004;8(4): 735–753.

Beutler E. Hemochromatosis: genetics and pathophysiology. *Annu Rev Med.* 2006;57:331–347.

Heeney MM, Andrews NC. Iron hemostasis and inherited iron overload disorders: an overview. *Hematol Clin North Am.* 2004;18(6):1379–1403.

Pietrangelo A. Hereditary hemochromatosis: a new look at an old disease. *NEJM.* 2004;350:2383–2397.

Powell LW. Hemochromatosis. In: Kasper D, Braunwald E, Fauci A, et al. eds. *Harrison's Principles of Internal Medicine.* 16th ed. McGraw-Hill; 2005.

Hemophilias

Aster JC. Red blood cell and bleeding disorders. In: Kumar V, Abbas AK, Fausto N. *Robbins and Cotran Pathologic Basis of Disease.* 7th ed. Elsevier Saunders; 2005.

Davie EW, Fujikawa K, Kisiel W. The coagulation cascade: initation, maintenance, and regulation. *Biochemistry.* 1991; 30(43):10363–10370.

Handin RI. Disorders of coagulation and thrombosis. In: Kasper D, Braunwald E, Fauci A, et al. eds. *Harrison's Principles of Internal Medicine.* 16th ed. McGraw-Hill; 2005.

Jagneaux T, Taylor DE, Kantrow SP. Coagulation in sepsis. *Am J Med Sci.* 2004;328(4):196–204.

Mannuci P, Tuddenham E. The hemophilias–from royal gene to gene therapy. *NEJM.* 200;344:1773–1779.

Hemostasis

Handin RI. Bleeding and thrombosis. In: Kasper D, Braunwald E, Fauci A, et al. eds. *Harrison's Principles of Internal Medicine.* 16th ed. McGraw-Hill; 2005.

Mitchell RN. Hemodynamic disorders, thromboembolic disease, and shock. In: Kumar V, Abbas AK, Fausto N. *Robbins and Cotran Pathologic Basis of Disease.* 7th ed. Elsevier Saunders; 2005.

Hepatitis B

Buccolo LS. *Clin Fam Pract.* 2005;7(1):105–125.

Ganem D, Prince AM. Hepatitis B virus infection—natural history and clinical consequences. *NEJM.* 2004;350:1118–1129.

Lin KW, Kirchner JT. Hepatitis B. *Am Fam Physician.* 2004; 69(1):75–82.

Mims C, Dockrell H, Goering R, et al. *Medical Microbiology.* 3rd ed. Elsevier Mosby Saunders; 2005.

Ocama P, Opio CK, Lee WM. Hepatitis B virus infection: current status. *Am J Med.* 2005;118(12):1413.e15–1413.e22.

Hepatitis C

Kim JD, Sherker AH. Antiviral therapy: role in the management of extrahepatic diseases. *Gastroenterol Clin North Am.* 2004;33:693–708.

Lauer GM, Walker BD. Hepatitis C virus infection. *NEJM.* 2001;345:41–52.

Patel K, Zekry A, McHutchinson JG. Steatosis and chronic hepatitis C virus infection: mechanisms and significance. *Clin Liver Dis.* 2005;9(3):399–410.

Pawlotsky JM. Pathophysiology of hepatitis C virus infection and related liver disease. *Trends Microbiol.* 2004;12(2):96–102.

Thomas DL, Seeff LB. Natural history hepatitis C. *Clin Liver Dis.* 2005;9(3):383–398.

Human Immunodeficiency Virus

CDC. 1993 Revised classification system for HIV infection and expanded surveillance case definition for AIDS among adolescents and adults. *MMWR.* 1992;41(RR-17).

Fauci AS, Lane HC. Human immunodeficiency virus disease: AIDS and related disorders. In: Kasper D, Braunwald E, Fauci A, et al. eds. *Harrison's Principles of Internal Medicine.* 16th ed. McGraw-Hill; 2005.

Fauci, AS. HIV and AIDS: 20 years of science. *Nat Med.* 2003; 9(7):703–839.

Kahn JO, Walker BD. Acute human immunodeficiency virus type 1 infection. *NEJM.* 1998;339:33–39.

Mims C, Dockrell H, Goering R, et al. *Medical Microbiology.* 3rd ed. Elsevier Mosby Saunders; 2005.

Murray PR, Rosenthal KS, Kobayashi GS, et al. *Medical Microbiology.* 4th ed. Mosby; 2002.

Picker LJ. Immunopathogenesis of acute AIDS virus infection. *Curr Opin Immunol.* 2006;18:399–405.

Rowland-Jones SL. AIDS pathogenesis what have two decades of HIV research taught us? *Nat Rev Immunol.* 2003;3:343–347.

Stebbing J, Gazzard B, Douek DC. Where does HIV live? *NEJM.* 2004;350:1872–1880.

Humoral Immunity

Janeway CA, Travers P, Walport M, et al. *Immunobiology: The Immune System in Health and Disease.* 5th ed. Garland Publishers; 2001.

Kindt TJ, Goldsby RA, Osborne BA, et al. *Kuby Immunology.* 6th ed. W.H. Freeman; 2007.

Parham P. *The Immune System.* Garland Publishers; 2000.

Huntington's Disease

Anderson KE. Huntington's disease and related disorders. *Psychiatr Clin North Am.* 2005;28(1):275–290.

Blumenfeld H. *Neuroanatomy through Clinical Cases. Sinauer;* 2002.

Caselli RJ, Boeve BF. The degenerative dementias. In: Goetz CG. *Textbook of Clinical Neurology.* 2nd ed. Elsevier; 2003.

Cattaneo E, Rigamonti D, Goffredo D. Loss of normal huntingtin function: new developments in Huntington's disease research. *Trends Neurosci.* 2001;24(3):182–188.

DeLong MR, Juncos JL. Parkinson's disease and other movement disorders. In: Kasper D, Braunwald E, Fauci A, et al. eds. *Harrison's Principles of Internal Medicine.* 16th ed. McGraw-Hill; 2005.

Gutekunst C, Norflus F, Hersch SM. Recent advances in Huntington's disease. *Curr Opin Neurol.* 2000;13(4):445–450.

HOPES: Huntington's outreach project for education, at Stanford. Causes of Huntington's Disease page. Available at: http://www.stanford.edu/group/hopes/causes/index/cshome. html. Accessed August 30, 2006.

Messing RO. Nervous system disorders. In: McPhee SJ, Lingappa VR, Ganong WF. *Pathophysiology of Disease.* 4th ed. McGraw-Hill; 2003.

Sharma N, Standaert DG. Inherited movement disorders. *Neurol Clin N Am.* 2002;20(3):759–778.

Hypercalcemia

Potts JT. Diseases of the parathyroid gland and other hyper- and hypocalcemic disorders. In: Kasper D, Braunwald E, Fauci A, et al. eds. *Harrison's Principles of Internal Medicine.* 16th ed. McGraw-Hill; 2005.

Shoback DM, Strewler GJ. Disorders of the parathyroids and calcium metabolism. In: McPhee SJ, Lingappa VR, Ganong WF. *Pathophysiology of Disease.* 4th ed. McGraw-Hill; 2003.

Hyperkalemia

Hollander-Rodriguez JC, Calvert JF. Hyperkalemia. *Am Fam Physician.* 2006;73(2):283–290.

Rose BD, Post TW. *Clinical Physiology of Acid-base and Electrolyte Disorders.* 5th ed. McGraw-Hill; 2000.

Schaefer TJ, Wolford RW. Disorders of potassium. *Emerg Med Clin N Am.* 2005;23:723–747.

Singer GG, Brenner BM. Fluid and electrolyte disturbances. In: Kasper D, Braunwald E, Fauci A, et al. eds. *Harrison's Principles of Internal Medicine.* 16th ed. McGraw-Hill; 2005.

Hypernatremia

Adrgoue HJ, Madias NE. Hypernatremia. *NEJM.* 2000;342: 1493–1499.

Fall PJ. Hyponatremia and hypernatremia. *J Postgrad Med [serial online].* May 2000;Vol. 107 No 5.

Lin M, Liu SJ, Lim IT. Disorders of water imbalance. *Emerg Med Clin Am.* 2005;23(3):749–770.

Hyperparathyroidism

Ahmad R, Hammon JM. Primary, secondary, and tertiary hyperparathyroidism. *Otolaryngol Clin North Am.* 2004; 37(4):701–713.

Bringhurst RF, Demay MB, Kronenberg HM. Hormones and disorders of mineral metabolism. In: Adashi EY, Aiello LP, Arnold A, et al. eds. *Larsen: Williams Textbook of Endocrinology.* 10th ed. Elsevier Saunders; 2003.

Khan A, Bilezikian J. Primary hyperparathyroidism: pathophysiology and impact on bone. *CMAJ.* 2000;163(2): 173–175.

Sherman SI, Gagel RF. Disorders affecting multiple endocrine systems. In: Kasper D, Braunwald E, Fauci A, et al. eds. *Harrison's Principles of Internal Medicine.* 16th ed. McGraw-Hill; 2005.

Hypersensitivity Reaction Type 1

Abbas AK. Diseases of immunity. In: Kumar V, Abbas AK, Fausto N. *Robbins and Cotran Pathologic Basis of Disease.* 7th ed. Elsevier Saunders; 2005.

Janeway CA, Travers P, Walport M, et al. *Immunobiology: The Immune System in Health and Disease.* 5th ed. Garland Publishers; 2001.

Kindt TJ, Goldsby RA, Osborne BA, et al. *Kuby Immunology.* 6th ed. W.H. Freeman; 2007.

Larson, K. *Hypersensitivities.* Philadelphia, PA: Drexel University College of Medicine; 2006.

Hypersensitivity Reaction Type 2

Abbas AK. Diseases of immunity. In: Kumar V, Abbas AK, Fausto N. *Robbins and Cotran Pathologic Basis of Disease,* 7th ed. Elsevier Saunders; 2005.

Janeway CA, Travers P, Walport M, et al. *Immunobiology: The Immune System in Health and Disease.* 5th ed. Garland Publishers; 2001.

Kindt TJ, Goldsby RA, Osborne BA et al. *Kuby Immunology.* 6th ed. W.H. Freeman; 2007.

Larson K. *Hypersensitivities.* Philadelphia. PA: Drexel University College of Medicine; 2006.

Hypersensitivity Reaction Type 3

Abbas AK. Diseases of immunity. In: Kumar V, Abbas AK, Fausto N. *Robbins and Cotran Pathologic Basis of Disease.* 7th ed. Elsevier Saunders; 2005.

Janeway CA, Travers P, Walport M, et al. *Immunobiology: The Immune System in Health and Disease.* 5th ed. Garland Publishers; 2001.

Kindt TJ, Goldsby RA, Osborne BA, et al. *Kuby Immunology.* 6th ed. W.H. Freeman; 2007.

Larson, K. *Hypersensitivities.* Philadelphia, PA: Drexel University College of Medicine; 2006.

Hypersensitivity Reaction Type 4

Abbas AK. Diseases of immunity. In: Kumar V, Abbas AK, Fausto N. *Robbins and Cotran Pathologic Basis of Disease.* 7th ed. Elsevier Saunders; 2005.

Janeway CA, Travers P, Walport M, et al. *Immunobiology: The Immune System in Health and Disease.* 5th ed. Garland Publishers; 2001.

Kindt TJ, Goldsby RA, Osborne BA, et al. *Kuby Immunology.* 6th ed. W.H. Freeman; 2007.

Larson K. *Hypersensitivities.* Philadelphia, PA: Drexel University College of Medicine; 2006.

Hypertension

Beevers G, Lip GY, O'Brien E. ABC of hypertension: the pathophysiology of hypertension. *BMJ.* 2001;322:912–916.

Fisher ND, Williams GH. Hypertensive vascular disease. In: Kasper D, Braunwald E, Fauci, A, et al. eds. *Harrison's Principles of Internal Medicine.* 16th ed. McGraw-Hill; 2005.

Ganong WF. Cardiovascular disorders: vascular disease. In: McPhee SJ, Lingappa VR, Ganong WF. *Pathophysiology of Disease.* 4th ed. McGraw-Hill; 2003.

Hyperthyroidism

Jameson JL, Weetman AP. Disorders of the thyroid gland. In: Kasper D, Braunwald E, Fauci A, et al. eds. *Harrison's Principles of Internal Medicine.* 16th ed. McGraw-Hill; 2005.

Maitra A, Abbas AK. The endocrine system. In: Kumar V, Abbas AK, Fausto N. *Robbins and Cotran Pathologic Basis of Disease.* 7th ed. Elsevier Saunders; 2005.

McPhee SJ, Bauer DC. Thyroid disease. In: McPhee SJ, Lingappa VR, Ganong WF. *Pathophysiology of Disease.* 4th ed. McGraw-Hill; 2003.

Hypocalcemia

Potts Jr JT. Diseases of the parathyroid gland and other hyper- and hypocalcemic disorders. In: Kasper D, Braunwald E, Fauci A, et al. eds. *Harrison's Principles of Internal Medicine.* 16th ed. McGraw-Hill; 2005.

Sarko J. Bone and mineral metabolism. *Emerg Med Clin North Am.* 2005;23(3):703–2.

Shoback DM, Strewler GJ. Disorders of the parathyroids and calcium metabolism. In: McPhee SJ, Lingappa VR, Ganong WF. *Pathophysiology of Disease.* 4th ed. McGraw-Hill; 2003.

Hypokalemia

Gennari FJ. Hypokalemia. *N Engl J Med* 1998;339:451–458.

Schaefer TJ, Wolford RW. Disorders of potassium. *Emerg Med Clin N Am.* 2005;23:723–747.

Singer GG, Brenner BM. Fluid and electrolyte disturbances. In: Kasper D, Braunwald E, Fauci A, et al. *Harrison's Principles of Internal Medicine.* 16th ed. McGraw-Hill; 2005.

Hyponatremia

Adrogué HJ, Madias NE. Hyponatremia. *NEJM.* 2000;342: 1581–1589.

Goh KP. Management of hyponatremia. *Am Fam Physician.* 2004;69(10):2387–2394.

Lin M, Liu SJ, Lim IT. Disorders of water imbalance. *Emerg Med Clin Am.* 2005;23(3):749–770.

Hypothyroidism

Jameson JL, Weetman AP. Disorders of the thyroid gland. In: Kasper D, Braunwald E, Fauci A, et al. eds. *Harrison's Principles of Internal Medicine.* 16th ed. McGraw-Hill; 2005.

McPhee SJ, Bauer DC. Thyroid disease. In: McPhee SJ, Lingappa VR, Ganong WF. *Pathophysiology of Disease.* 4th ed. McGraw-Hill; 2003.

Larsen PR, Davies TF, Schlumberger M, et al. Thyroid physiology and diagnostic evaluation of patients with thyroid disorders. In: Adashi EY, Aiello LP, Arnold A, et al. eds. *Larsen: Williams Textbook of Endocrinology.* 10th ed. Elsevier Saunders; 2003.

Infective Endocarditis

Bloch KC. Infectious diseases. In: McPhee SJ, Lingappa VR, Ganong WF. *Pathophysiology of Disease.* 4th ed. McGraw-Hill; 2003.

Crawford MH, Durack DT. Clinical presentation of infective endocarditis. *Cardiol Clin.* 2003;21:159–166.

Mylonakis E, Calderwood SB. Infective endocarditis in adults. *NEJM.* 2001;345:1318–1330.

Fowler Jr. VG, Scheld WM, Bayer AS. Endocarditis and intravascular infections. In: Mandell, Bennett, & Dolin: *Principles and Practice of Infectious Diseases.* 6th ed. Churchill Livingstone/Elsevier, 2005.

Karchmer AW. Infective endocarditis. In: Kasper D, Braunwald E, Fauci A, et al. eds. *Harrison's Principles of Internal Medicine.* 16th ed. McGraw-Hill; 2005.

Moreillon P, Que Y. Infective endocarditis. *Lancet.* 2004;363 (9403):139–149.

Intracranial Hemorrhage

Blumenfeld H. *Neuroanatomy through Clinical Cases.* Sinauer; 2002.

Chung C, Caplan LR. Neurovascular disorders. In: Goetz CG. *Textbook of Clinical Neurology.* 2nd ed. Elsevier; 2003.

Messing RO. Nervous system diseases. In: McPhee SJ, Lingappa VR, Ganong WF. *Pathophysiology of Disease.* 4th ed. McGraw-Hill; 2003.

Smith WS, Johnston SC, Easton JD. Cerebrovascular diseases. In: Kasper D, Braunwald E, Fauci A, et al. eds. *Harrison's Principles of Internal Medicine.* 16th ed. McGraw-Hill; 2005.

Iron Deficiency Anemia

Davoren JB. Blood disorders. In: McPhee SJ, Lingappa VR, Ganong WF. *Pathophysiology of Disease.* 4th ed. McGraw-Hill; 2003.

Heeney MM, Andrews NC. Iron homeostasis and inherited iron overload disorders: an overview. *Hematol Oncol Clin N Am.* 2004;18(6):1379–1403.

Smith CM, Marks AD, Lieberman MA, et al. eds. *Marks' Basic Medical Biochemistry: A Clinical Approach.* Lippincott Williams & Wilkins; 1996.

Ischemic Stroke

Blumenfeld H. *Neuroanatomy through Clinical Cases.* Sinauer; 2002.

Frosch MP, Anthony DC, De Girolami U. The central nervous system. In: Kumar V, Abbas AK, Fausto N, eds. *Robbins and Cotran Pathologic Basis of Disease.* 7th ed. Elsevier Saunders; 2005.

Kothari RU, Crocco TJ, Barsan WG. Stroke. In: Marx: *Rosen's Emergency Medicine: Concepts and Clinical Practice.* 6th ed. Mosby, 2006.

Messing RO. Nervous system diseases. In: McPhee SJ, Lingappa VR, Ganong WF. *Pathophysiology of Disease.* 4th ed. McGraw-Hill; 2003.

Smith WS, Johnston SC, Easton JD. Cerebrovascular diseases. In: Kasper D, Braunwald E, Fauci A, et al. *Harrison's Principles of Internal Medicine.* 16th ed. McGraw-Hill; 2005.

Lymphoid Leukemia and Lymphomas

Armitage JO, Longo DL. Malignancies of lymphoid cells. In: Kasper D, Braunwald E, Fauci A, et al. eds. *Harrison's Principles of Internal Medicine.* 16th ed. McGraw-Hill; 2005.

Aster JC. Diseases of white blood cells, lymph nodes, spleen, and thymus. In: Kumar V, Abbas AK, Fausto N. *Robbins and Cotran Pathologic Basis of Disease.* 7th ed. Elsevier Saunders; 2005.

Tripathy D, Rubenstein J. Neoplasia. In: McPhee SJ , Lingappa VR, Ganong WF. *Pathophysiology of Disease.* 4th ed. McGraw-Hill; 2003.

Meningitis

Roos KL, Tyler KL. Meningitis, encephalitis, brain abscess, and empyema. In: Kasper D, Braunwald E, Fauci A, et al. *Harrison's Principles of Internal Medicine.* 16th ed. McGraw-Hill; 2005.

Losh DP. Central nervous system infections. *Clin Fam Pract.* 2004;6(1):1–17.

Tunkel, AR. Central nervous system infections. In: Mandell, Bennett, & Dolin: *Principles and Practice of Infectious Diseases.* 6th ed. Elsevier Saunders; 2005.

van de Beek D, de Gans J, Tunkel AR, Wijdicks EFM Community-acquired bacterial meningitis in adults. *N Engl J Med.* 2006;354:44–53.

Menopause

Boron W, Boulpaep E. Medical *Physiology: A Cellular and Molecular Approach.* Elsevier Saunders; 2005.

Carr BR, Bradshaw KD. Disorders of the ovary and female reproductive tract. In: Kasper D, Braunwald E, Fauci A, et al. eds. *Harrison's Principles of Internal Medicine.* 16th ed. McGraw-Hill; 2005.

Lingappa VR Disorders of the female reproductive tract. In: McPhee SJ, Lingappa VR, Ganong WF. *Pathophysiology of Disease.* 4th ed. McGraw-Hill; 2003.

Rosen M, Cedars MI. Female reproductive endocrinology & infertility. In: Greenspan FS, Gardner DG. *Basic and Clinical Endocrinology.* 7th ed. McGraw-Hill; 2004.

Stenchever MA, Droegemueller W, Herbst AL, et al. *Comprehensive Gynecology.* 4th ed. Mosby; 2001.

Wilson MM. Menopause. *Clin Geriatr Med* 2003;19:483–506.

Metabolic Acidosis

Anesthesia Education Website. Acid-base physiology page. Available at http://www.anesthesiamcq.com/default.php. Accessed April 16, 2006.

Casaletto JJ. Differential diagnosis of metabolic acidosis. *Emerg Med Clin N Am.* 2005;23:771–787.

DuBose Jr TD. Acid-base disorders. In: *Brenner & Rector's The Kidney.* 7th ed. Elsevier Saunders; 2004.

Myers AR. *National Medical Series for Independent Study: Medicine.* 5th ed. Lippincott Williams & Wilkins; 2005.

Rose BD, Post TW. *Clinical Physiology of Acid-Base and Electrolyte Disorders.* 5th ed. McGraw-Hill; 2001.

Metabolic Alkalosis

Anesthesia Education Website. Acid-base physiology page. Available at http://www.anaesthesiamcq.com/default.php. Accessed April 16, 2006.

DuBose Jr. TD. Acid-base disorders. In: *Brenner & Rector's The Kidney.* 7th ed. Elsevier Saunders; 2004.

Galla JH. Metabolic alkalosis. *J Am Soc Nephrol.* 2000;11(2): 369–376.

Kellum JA. Determinants of plasma acid-base balance. *Crit Care Clin.* 2005;21:329–346.

Rose BD, Post TW. *Clinical Physiology of Acid-base and Electrolyte Disorders.* 5th ed. McGraw-Hill; 2001.

Multiple Sclerosis

Bar-Or A. Immunology of multiple sclerosis. *Neurol Clin.* 2005;23:149–175.

Bjartmar C, Trapp BD. Axonal and neuronal degeneration in multiple sclerosis: mechanisms and functional consequences. *Curr Opin Neurol.* 2001;14(3):271–278.

Frohman EM, Racke MK, Raine CS. Multiple sclerosis–the plaque and its pathogenesis. *NEJM.* 2006;354: 942–955.

Hauser SL, Goodin DS. Multiple sclerosis and other demyelinating diseases. In: Kasper D, Braunwald E, Fauci A, et al. *Harrison's Principles of Internal Medicine.* 16th ed. McGraw-Hill; 2005.

Lucchinetti C, Bruck W, Noseworthy J. Multiple sclerosis: recent developments in neuropathology, pathogenesis, magnetic resonance imaging studies and treatment. *Curr Opin Neurol.* 2001;14(3):259–269.

Lucchinetti CF, Parisi J, Bruck W. The pathology of multiple sclerosis. *Neurol Clin.* 2005;23:77–105.

Noseworthy JH, Lucchinetti C, Rodriguez M, et al. Multiple sclerosis. *NEJM.* 2000;343:938–952.

Sorensen PS. Multiple sclerosis: pathophysiology revisited. *Lancet Neurol.* 2005;4(1):9–10.

Myasthenia Gravis

Bartt R, Shannon KM. Autoimmune and inflammatory disorders. In: Goetz CG. *Textbook of Clinical Neurology.* 2nd ed. Elsevier Saunders; 2003.

Drachman DB. Myasthenia gravis and other diseases of the neuromuscular junction. In: Kasper D, Braunwald E, Fauci A, et al. *Harrison's Principles of Internal Medicine.* 16th ed. McGraw-Hill; 2005.

Hughes BW, De Casillas ML, Kaminski HJ. Pathophysiology of myasthenia gravis. *Sem Neurol.* 2004;24(1):21–30.

Messing RO. Nervous system disorders. In: McPhee SJ, Lingappa VR, Ganong WF. *Pathophysiology of Disease.* 4th ed. McGraw-Hill; 2003.

Myeloid Leukemia and Lymphomas

Hughes BW, De Casillas ML, Kaminski HJ. Pathophysiology of myasthenia gravis. *Sem Neurol.* 2004;24(1):21–30.

Longo DL, Anderson KC. Multiple myeloma In: Kasper D, Braunwald E, Fauci A, et al. eds. *Harrison's Principles of Internal Medicine.* 16th ed. McGraw-Hill; 2005.

Tripathy D, Rubenstein J. Neoplasia. In: McPhee SJ, Lingappa VR, Ganong WF. *Pathophysiology of Disease.* 4th ed. McGraw-Hill; 2003.

Wetzler M, Byrd JC, Bloomfield CD. Acute and chronic myeloid leukemia. In: Kasper D, Braunwald E, Fauci A, et al. eds. *Harrison's Principles of Internal Medicine.* 16th ed. McGraw-Hill; 2005.

Myocardial Ischemia and Infarction

Antman EM, Braunwald E. ST-segment elevation myocardial infarction. In: Kasper D, Braunwald E, Fauci A, et al. eds. *Harrison's Principles of Internal Medicine.* 16th ed. McGraw-Hill; 2005.

Cannon CP, Braunwald E. Unstable angina and non-ST-elevation myocardial infarction. In: Kasper D, Braunwald E, Fauci A, et al. eds. *Harrison's Principles of Internal Medicine.* 16th ed. McGraw-Hill; 2005.

Hughes BW, De Casillas ML, Kaminski HJ. Pathophysiology of myasthenia gravis. *Sem Neurol.* 2004;24(1):21–30.

Lilly L, ed. *Pathophysiology of Heart Disease: A Collaborative Project of Medical Students and Faculty.* 3rd ed. Lippincott Williams & Wilkins; 2003.

Selwyn AP, Braunwald E. Ischemic heart disease. In: Kasper D, Braunwald E, Fauci A, et al. eds. *Harrison's Principles of Internal Medicine.* 16th ed. McGraw-Hill; 2005.

Nephrolithiasis

Asplin JR, Coe FL, Favus MJ. Nephrolithiasis. In: Kasper D, Braunwald E, Fauci A, et al. eds. *Harrison's Principles of Internal Medicine.* 16th ed. McGraw-Hill; 2005.

Balaji K, M Menon. Urolithiasis: mechanism of stone formation. *Urol Clin North Am.* 1997;24(1).

Coe FL, Evan A, Worcester E. Kidney stone disease. *J Clin Invest* 2005;115(10):2598–2608.

Coe FL, Favus MJ, Asplin JR. Nephrolithiasis. In: Brenner BM. *Brenner & Rector's The Kidney.* 7th ed. Elsevier Saunders; 2004.

Coe FL, Evan A, Worcester E. Kidney stone disease. *J Clin Invest.* 2005;115(10):2598–2608.

Moe OW. Kidney stones: pathophysiology and medical management. *Lancet.* 2006;367(9507):333–344 .

Pak CY. Kidney stones. *Lancet.* 1998;351:1797–1801.

Nephrotic Syndrome

Brady HR, O'Meara YM, Brenner BM. Glomerular diseases. In: Kasper D, Braunwald E, Fauci A, et al. eds. *Harrison's Principles of Internal Medicine.* 16th ed. McGraw-Hill; 2005.

Brenner & Rector's The Kidney. 7th ed. Elsevier Saunders; 2004.

Hamm LL, Batuman V. Edema in the nephrotic syndrome: new aspect of an old enigma. *J Am Soc Nephrol.* 2003; 14(12):3288–3289.

Hogg RJ. Adolescents with proteinuria and/or the nephrotic syndrome. *Adolesc Med Clin.* 2005;16(1):163–172.

Orth SR, Ritz E. The nephrotic syndrome. *NEJM.* 1998;338: 1202–1211.

Osteoarthritis

Aigner T, McKenna L. Molecular pathology and pathobiology of osteoarthritic cartilage. *Cell Mol Life Sci.* 2002;59(1):5–18.

Brandt KD. Osteoarthritis. In: Kasper D, Braunwald E, Fauci A, et al. *Harrison's Principles of Internal Medicine.* 16th ed. McGraw-Hill; 2005.

Manek N, Lane N. Osteoarthritis: current concepts in diagnosis and management. *Am Fam Physician.* 2000;61:1795–1804.

Rosenberg AE. Bones, joints, and soft tissue tumors. In: Kumar V, Abbas AK, Fausto N, eds. *Robbins and Cotran Pathologic Basis of Disease.* 7th ed. Elsevier Saunders; 2005.

Osteomalacia

Bringhurst FR, Demay MB, Kronenberg HM. Hormones and disorders of mineral metabolism. In: Adashi EY, Aiello LP, Arnold A, et al. eds. *Larsen: Williams Textbook of Endocrinology.* 10th ed. Elsevier Saunders; 2003.

Pettifor JM. Rickets and vitamin D deficiency in children and adolescents. *Endocrinol Metab Clin N Am.* 2005;34: 537–553.

Rosenberg AE. Bones, joints, and soft tissue tumors. In: Kumar V, Abbas AK, Fausto N. eds. *Robbins and Cotran Pathologic Basis of Disease.* 7th ed. Elsevier Saunders; 2005.

Shoback DM, Strewler GJ. Disorders of the parathyroids and calcium metabolism. In: McPhee SJ, Lingappa VR, Ganong WF. *Pathophysiology of Disease.* 4th ed. McGraw-Hill; 2003.

Osteoporosis

Lindsay R, Cosman F. Osteoporosis. In: Kasper D, Braunwald E, Fauci A, et al. eds. *Harrison's Principles of Internal Medicine.* 16th ed. McGraw-Hill; 2005.

Pathophysiology of osteoporosis (module 3). In AMA Osteoporosis Management: the Online series. Available at: http://www.ama-cmeonline.com/osteo_mgmt/. Accessed November 8, 2006.

Pancreatitis

Greenberger NJ, Toskes PP. Acute and chronic pancreatitis. In: Kasper D, Braunwald E, Fauci A, et al. eds. *Harrison's Priciples of Internal Medicine.* 16th ed. McGraw-Hill; 2005.

McPhee SJ. Disorders of the exocrine pancreas. In: McPhee SJ, Lingappa VR, Ganong WF. *Pathophysiology of Disease.* 4th ed. McGraw-Hill; 2003.

Sreer ML, Waxman I, Freedman S. Chronic pancreatitis. *NEJM.* 1995;332:1482–1490.

Sreinburg W, Tenner S. Acute pancreatitis. *NEJM.* 1994; 330(17):1198–1210.

Parkinson's Disease

Blumenfeld H. *Neuroanatomy through Clinical Cases.* Sinauer; 2002.

Delong MR, Juncos JL. Parkinson's disease and other movement disorders. In: Kasper D, Braunwald E, Fauci A, et al. eds. *Harrison's Priciples of Internal Medicine.* 16th ed. McGraw-Hill; 2005

Jenner P, Olanow CW. The pathogenesis of cell death in Parkinson's disease. *Neurology.* 2006:66(suppl4): S24–S36.

Messing RO. Nervous system disorders. In: McPhee SJ, Lingappa VR, Ganong WF. *Pathophysiology of Disease.* 4th ed. McGraw-Hill; 2003.

Moore DJ, West AB, Dawson VL, Dawson TM. Molecular pathophysiology of Parkinson's disease. *Annu Rev Neurosci.* 2005;28:57–87.

Schapira AHV. Etiology of Parkinson's disease. *Neurology.* 2006;66(suppl4):S10–S23.

Polycystic Ovary Syndrome

Adams JM, Taylor AE, Crowley WF, et al. Polycystic ovarian morphology with regular ovulatory cycles: insights in the pathophysiology of polycystic ovarian syndrome. *J Clin Endocrinol Metab.* 2004;89(9):4343–4350.

Balen A. The pathophysiology of polycystic ovarian syndrome: trying to understand PCOS and its endocrinology. *Best Pract Res Clin Obstet Gynaecol.* 2004;18(5):685–706.

Buggs C, Rosenfield RL. Polycystic ovarian syndrome in adolescence. *Endocrinol Metab Clin N Am.* 2005;34:677–705.

Ehrmann, DA. Polycystic ovarian syndrome. *NEJM.* 2005; 352:1223–1236

Purcell KJ, Lingappa VR, Taylor RN. Disorders of the female reproductive tract. In: McPhee SJ, Lingappa VR, Ganong WF. *Pathophysiology of Disease.* 4th ed. McGraw-Hill; 2003.

Serdar E. Bulun Adashi EY. The physiology and pathology of the female reproductive axis. In: Adashi EY, Aiello LP, Arnold A, et al. eds. *Larsen: Williams Textbook of Endocrinology.* 10th ed. Elsevier Saunders; 2003.

Stenchever MA, Droegemueller W, Herbst AL, et al. Hyperandrogenism. In: *Stenchever: Comprehensive Gynecology.* 4th ed. Mosby; 2001.

Platelet Disorders

Aster JC. Red blood cell and bleeding disorders. In: Kumar V, Abbas AK, Fausto N. *Robbins and Cotran Pathologic Basis of Disease.* 7th ed. Elsevier Saunders; 2005.

Handin RI. Disorders of the platelet and vessel wall. In: Kasper D, Braunwald E, Fauci A, et al. eds. *Harrison's Principles of Internal Medicine.* 16th ed. McGraw-Hill; 2005.

Mannucci PM, Tuddenham E. The hemophilias—from royal gene to gene therapy. *NEJM.* 2001;344:1773–1779.

Mannucci PM. Treatment of von Willebrand's disease. *NEJM.* 2004;351:683–694.

Pneumonia

Alcon A, Fabregas N, Torres A. Pathophysiology of pneumonia. *Clin Chest Med.* 2005;26:39–46.

Bloch KC. Infectious Diseases. In: McPhee SJ, Lingappa VR, Ganong WF. *Pathophysiology of Disease.* 4th ed. McGraw-Hill; 2003.

Husain AN, Kumar V. The lung. In: Kumar V, Abbas AK, Fausto N, eds. *Robbins and Cotran Pathologic Basis of Disease.* 7th ed. Elsevier Saunders; 2005.

Marrie TJ, Campbell AD, Walker DH, Low DE. Pneumonia. In: Kasper D, Braunwald E, Fauci A, et al. eds. *Harrison's Priciples of Internal Medicine.* 16th ed. McGraw-Hill; 2005.

Preeclampsia Eclampsia

Beckmann CR. *Obstetrics and Gynecology.* 4th ed. Lippincott Williams & Wilkins; 2002.

Davison JM, Homuth V, Jeyabalan A, et al. New aspects in the pathophysiology of preeclampsia. *J Am Soc Nephrol.* 2004; 15:2440–2448.

Sibai BM. Hypertension. In: Gabbe SG, Niebyl JR, Simpson JL. *Obstetrics–Normal and Problem Pregnancies.* 4th ed. Churchill Linvingstone; 2002.

Primary Hypercoagulable States

Davie EW, Fujikawa K, Kisiel W. The coagulation cascade: initiation, maintenance, and regulation. *Biochemistry.* 1991;30(43):10363–10370.

Davoren JB. Blood disorders. In: McPhee SJ, Lingappa VR, Ganong WF. *Pathophysiology of Disease.* 4th ed. McGraw-Hill; 2003.

Feero W. Genetic thrombophilia. *Prim Care Clin Office* Pract. 2004;31:685–709.

Handin RI. Disorders of coagulation and thrombosis. In: Kasper D, Braunwald E, Fauci A, et al. eds. *Harrison's Principles of Internal Medicine.* 16th ed. McGraw-Hill; 2005.

Jagneaux T, Taylor DE, Kantrow SP. Coagulation in sepsis. *Am J Med Sci.* 2004;328(4):196–204.

Levine JS, Branch DW, Rauch J. The antiphospholipid syndrome. *NEJM.* 2002;346;752–763.

Mitchell RN. Hemodynamic disorders, thromboembolic disease, and shock. In: Kumar V, Abbas AK, Fausto N. *Robbins and Cotran Pathologic Basis of Disease.* 7th ed. Elsevier Saunders; 2005.

Nachman RL, Silverstein R. Hypercoagulable states. *Ann Intern Med.* 1993;119(8):819–827.

Primary Immune Deficiencies

Abbas AK. Diseases of immunity. In: Kumar V, Abbas AK, Fausto N. *Robbins and Cotran Pathologic Basis of Disease.* 7th ed. Elsevier Saunders; 2005.

Cooper MA, Pommering TL, Korany K. Primary immunodeficiencies. *Am Fam Physician.* 2003;68(10):2001–2010.

Cooper MS, Schroeder Jr HW, Primary immune defiency diseases. In: Kasper D, Braunwald E, Fauci A, et al. eds. *Harrison's Priciples of Internal Medicine.* 16th ed. McGraw-Hill; 2005.

Shames RS, Kishiyama JL. Disorders of the immune system. In: McPhee SJ, Lingappa VR, Ganong WF. *Pathophysiology of Disease.* 4th ed. McGraw-Hill; 2003.

Pulmonary Embolism

Boron W, Boulpaep E. *Medical Physiology: A Cellular and Molecular Approach.* Elsevier. Saunders; 2005.

Dalen JE. Pulmonary embolism: what have we learned since virchow? natural history, pathophysiology, and diagnosis. *Chest.* 2002;122:1440–1456.

Fedullo PF, Morris TA. Pulmonary thromboembolism. In: Mason RJ, Murray JF, Broaddus VC, et al. eds. *Murray & Nadel's Textbook of Respiratory Medicine.* 4th ed. Saunders; 2005.

Goldhaber SZ, Elliott CG. Acute pulmonary embolism: part I. *Circulation.* 2003;108:2726–2729.

Goldhaber SZ. Pulmonary embolism. *NEJM.* 1998;339(2): 93–106.

Kline JA, Runyon MS. Pulmonary embolism and deep venous thrombosis. In: Marx JA, Hockberger RS, Walls RM, et al. eds. *Rosen's Emergency Medicine: Concepts and Clinical Practice.* 5th ed. Mosby; 2002.

Prendergast TJ. Ruoss SJ. Pulmonary diseases. In: McPhee SJ, Lingappa VR, Ganong WF. *Pathophysiology of Disease.* 4th ed. McGraw-Hill; 2003.

Smulders YM. Pathophysiology and treatment of hemodynamic instability in acute pulmonary embolism: the pivotal role of pulmonary vasoconstriction. *Cardiovasc Res.* 2000; 48:23–33.

Renin-Angiotensin-Aldosterone System

Boron W, Boulpaep E. *Medical Physiology: A Cellular and Molecular Approach.* Elsevier Saunders; 2005.

Candido R, Burrell LM, Jandelait-Dahm K. Vasoactive peptides and the kidney. In: *Brenner & Rector's The Kidney.* 7th ed. Sauders; 2004.

Respiratory Acidosis

Anesthesia Education Website. Acid-base physiology page. Available at http://www.anaesthesiamcq.com/default.php. Accessed April 16, 2006.

Rose BD, Post TW. *Clinical Physiology of Acid-base and Electrolyte Disorders.* 5th ed. McGraw-Hill; 2000.

Respiratory Alkalosis

Anesthesia Education Website. Acid-base physiology page. Available at http://www.anaesthesiamcq.com/default.php. Accessed April 16, 2006.

Rose BD, Post TW. *Clinical Physiology of Acid-base and Electrolyte Disorders.* 5th ed. McGraw-Hill; 2000.

Rheumatoid Arthritis

Choy EH, Panayi GS. Cytokine pathways and joint inflammation in rheumatoid arthritis. *NEJM.* 2001;344(12): 907–916.

Rosenberg AE. Bones, joints, and soft tissue tumors. In: Kumar V, Abbas AK, Fausto N. eds. *Robbins and Cotran Pathologic Basis of Disease.* 7th ed. Elsevier Saunders; 2005.

Smith JB, Haynes MK. Rheumatod arthritis-a molecular understanding. *Ann Int Med.* 2002;136(12):908–922.

Sarcoidosis

Crystal RG. Sarcoidosis. In: Kasper D, Braunwald E, Fauci A, et al. *Harrison's Priciples of Internal Medicine.* 16th ed. McGraw-Hill; 2005.

Husain AN, Kumar V. The lung. In: Kumar V, Abbas AK, Fausto N. eds. *Robbins and Cotran Pathologic Basis of Disease.* 7th ed. Elsevier Saunders; 2005.

Maize JC, McCalmont TH. Diseases of the skin. In: McPhee SJ, Lingappa VR, Ganong WF. *Pathophysiology of Disease.* 4th ed. McGraw-Hill; 2003.

Sepsis Syndromes

Aird W. Sepsis and coagulation. *Crit Care Clin.* 2005;21: 417–431.

Aird WC. The role of the endothelium in severe sepsis and multiple organ dysfunction syndrome. *Blood.* 2003;101: 3765–3777.

Bloch KC. Infectious diseases. In: McPhee SJ, Lingappa VR, Ganong WF. *Pathophysiology of Disease.* 4th ed. McGraw-Hill; 2003.

Diehl JL, Borgel D. Sepsis and coagulation. *Curr Opin Crit Care.* 2005;11:454–460.

Hotchkiss RS, Karl IE. The pathophysiology and treatment of sepsis. *NEJM.* 2003;348(2):135–149.

Jacobi, J. Pathophysiology of sepsis. *Am J Health Syst Pharm.* 2002;59(4):S3–S8.

LaRosa SP. Sepsis: menu of new approaches replaces one therapy for all. *Cleve Clin J Med.* 2002;69(1):65–73.

Levy MM, Fink MP, Marshall JC, et al. 2001 SCCM/ESICM/ ACCP/ATS/SIS International Sepsis Definitions Conference. *Crit Care Med.* 2003;31(4):1250–1256.

Mumford RS. Severe sepsis and septic shock. In: Kasper D, Braunwald E, Fauci A, et al. eds. *Harrison's Priciples of Internal Medicine.* 16th ed. McGraw-Hill; 2005.

Nimah M, Brilli RJ. Coagulation dysfunction in sepsis and multiple organ system failure. *Crit Care Clin.* 2003;19: 441–458.

Syndrome of Inappropriate Antidiuretic Hormone Secretion

Adroque HJ, Madias NE. Hyponatremia. *NEJM.* 2000;342 (21):1581–1589.

Berl T, Verbalis J. Pathophysiology of water metabolism. In: *Brenner & Rector's The Kidney.* 7th ed. Saunders; 2004.

Robertson GL. Disorders of the neurohypopysis. In: Kasper D, Braunwald E, Fauci A, et al. eds. *Harrison's Priciples of Internal Medicine*. 16th ed. McGraw-Hill; 2005.

Rose BD, Post TW. *Clinical Physiology of Acid-base and Electrolyte Disorders*. 5th ed. McGraw-Hill; 2000.

Sickle Cell Anemia

Aster J. Red blood cell and bleeding disorders. In: Kumar V, Abbas AK, Fausto N. et al. eds. *Robbins and Cotran Pathologic Basis of Disease*. 7th ed. Elsevier Saunders; 2005.

Benz EJ. Hemoglobinopathies. In: Kasper D, Braunwald E, Fauci A, et al. *Harrison's Priciples of Internal Medicine*. 16th ed. McGraw-Hill; 2005.

Hebbel RP. Pathobiology of sickle cell disease. In: *Hoffman: Hematology: Basic Principles and Practice*. 4th ed. Curchill Livingstone; 2005.

Systemic Lupus Erythematosus

Abbas AK. Disease of immunity. In: Kumar V, Abbas AK, Fausto N. *Robbins and Cotran Pathologic Basis of Disease*. 7th ed. Elsevier Saunders; 2005.

Greidinger EL, Rosen A. Inflammatory rheumatic diseases. In: McPhee SJ, Lingappa VR, Ganong WF. *Pathophysiology of Disease*. 4th ed. McGraw-Hill; 2003.

Hahn BH. Systemic lupus erythematosus In: Kasper D, Braunwald E, Fauci A, et al. eds. *Harrison's Priciples of Internal Medicine*. 16th ed. McGraw-Hill; 2005.

Myers AR. *National Medical Series for Independent Study: Medicine*. 5th ed. Lippincott Williams & Wilkins; 2005.

Thrombocytopenia

Aster JC. Red blood cell and bleeding disorders. In: Kumar V, Abbas AK, Fausto N. eds. *Robbins and Cotran Pathologic Basis of Disease*. 7th ed. Elsevier Saunders; 2005.

Drew R. Critical issues in hematology: anemia, thrombocytopenia, coagulopathy, and blood product transfusions in critically ill patients. *Clin Chest Med*. 2003;24:607–622.

Handin RI. Disorders of the platelet and vessel wall. In: Kasper D, Braunwald E, Fauci A, et al. eds. *Harrison's Priciples of Internal Medicine*. 16th ed. McGraw-Hill; 2005.

Myers AR. *National Medical Series for Independent Study: Medicine*. 5th ed. Lippincott Williams & Wilkins; 2005.

Tortora GJ, Grabowski SR. *Principles of Anatomy and Physiology*. 9th ed. Wiley; 2000.

Tuberculosis

Goldberg S. Tuberculosis. *Clin Fam Pract*. 2004;6(1):175–197.

Infectious Disease Society of America. Diagnostic classification of TB. *Am J Respir Crit Care Med*. 2000;161(4):1376–1395.

McAdam A, Sharpe A. Infectiouse diseases. In: Kumar V, Abbas AK, Fausto N. eds. *Robbins and Cotran Pathologic Basis of Disease*. 7th ed. Elsevier Saunders; 2005.

Raviglione MC, O'Brien Tuberculosis RJ. In: Kasper D, Braunwald E, Fauci A, et al. eds. *Harrison's Priciples of Internal Medicine*. 16th ed. McGraw-Hill; 2005.

Tufariello JA, Chan J, Flynn JL. Latent tuberculosis: mechanisms of host and bacillus that contribute to persistent infection. *Lancet Infect Dis*. 2003;3(6):578–590.

Ulcerative Colitis

Friedman S, Blumberg RS. Inflammatory bowel disease. In: Kasper D, Braunwald E, Fauci A, et al. *Harrison's Priciples of Internal Medicine*. 16th ed. McGraw-Hill; 2005.

Jewell DP. Ulcerative colitis. In: Feldman: Sleisenger & Fortran's Gastrointestinal and Liver Disease. 7th ed. Saunders; 2002.

Podolsky DK. Inflammatory bowel disease. *NEJM*. 2002; 347:417–429.

Urinary Tract Infection

Alpers C. The kidney. In: Kumar V, Abbas AK, Fausto N. *Robbins and Cotran Pathologic Basis of Disease*. 7th ed. Elsevier Saunders; 2005.

Tolkoff-Rubin NE, Cotran RS, Rubin RH. Urinary tract infection, pyelnonephritis, and reflux nephropathy. In: *Brenner & Rector's The Kidney*. 7th ed. Saunders; 2004.

Valvular Regurgitation

Braunwald E. Valvular heart disease. In: Kasper D, Braunwald E, Fauci A, et al. eds. *Harrison's Priciples of Internal Medicine*. 16th ed. McGraw-Hill; 2005.

Kusumoto F. Cardiovascular disorders: heart disease. In: McPhee SJ, Lingappa VR, Ganong WF. *Pathophysiology of Disease*. 4th ed. McGraw-Hill; 2003.

Yachimski P, Lilly LS. Valvular heart disease. *Lilly Pathophysiology of Heart Disease: A Collaborative Project of Medical Students and Faculty*. 3rd ed. Lippincott Williams & Wilkins; 2003.

Valvular Stenosis

Braunwald E. Valvular heart disease. In: Kasper D, Braunwald E, Fauci A, et al. *Harrison's Priciples of Internal Medicine*. 16th ed. McGraw-Hill; 2005.

Kusumoto F. Cardiovascular disorders: heart disease. In: McPhee SJ, Lingappa VR, Ganong WF. *Pathophysiology of Disease*. 4th ed. McGraw-Hill; 2003.

Yachimski P, Lilly LS. Valvular heart disease. *Lilly Pathophysiology of Heart Disease: A Collaborative Project of Medical Students and Faculty*. 3rd ed. Lippincott Williams & Wilkins; 2003.

Vitamin B12 Deficiency

Aster JC. Red blood cell and bleeding disorders. In: Kumar V, Abbas AK, Fausto N, eds. *Robbins and Cotran Pathologic Basis of Disease*. 7th ed. Elsevier Saunders; 2005

Toh BH , van Driel IR, Gleeson, PA. Pernicious anemia. *NEJM*. 1997;337(20):1441–1448.

INDEX